One Virus, Two Countries

One Virus, Two Countries

What Covid-19 tells us about South Africa

STEVEN FRIEDMAN

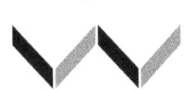

Published in South Africa by:
Wits University Press
1 Jan Smuts Avenue
Johannesburg 2001

www.witspress.co.za

Copyright © Steven Friedman 2021
Published edition © Wits University Press 2021

First published 2021

http://dx.doi.org.10.18772/12021117434

978-1-77614-743-4 (Paperback)
978-1-77614-744-1 (Hardback)
978-1-77614-745-8 (Web PDF)
978-1-77614-746-5 (EPUB)

All rights reserved. No part of this publication may be reproduced, stored in a retrieval system, or transmitted in any form or by any means, electronic, mechanical, photocopying, recording or otherwise, without the written permission of the publisher, except in accordance with the provisions of the Copyright Act, Act 98 of 1978.

Project manager: Catherine Damerell
Copy editor: Lee Smith
Proofreader: Tessa Botha
Indexer: Marlene Burger
Cover design: Hybrid Creative
Typeset in 11.5 point Minion Pro

CONTENTS

PREFACE	vii
LIST OF ACRONYMS	xiii
INTRODUCTION	1
CHAPTER 1 One Country, Two Realities	13
CHAPTER 2 Following the Science	25
CHAPTER 3 The Science Unravels	57
CHAPTER 4 The Blank Cheque	91
CHAPTER 5 The Path Not Taken	119
NOTES	133
REFERENCES	155
INDEX	175

PREFACE

Why take seriously a book on a pandemic written by a student of politics who has never studied medicine?

One of the mantras of South Africa's official response to Covid-19 (and that of many other countries) was that we should respond to the virus by 'following the science'. While this was an understandable response to an earlier failure to take science seriously – the government's response to HIV and Aids during the early years of the twenty-first century – it created its own problems, chief among them the assumption that there is an undisputed 'science' of Covid-19 which is available only to medical scientists – 'experts' who are, therefore, infallible messengers of the revealed truth. This too was central to the way in which the country's elites first responded to the disease. It ensured a slavish reverence for medical scientists, even when their claims appeared to ignore evidence available in the daily news, or were proved to be simply wrong, and served largely to close down public debate on the government's medical response to the virus. And, while some scientists complained incessantly that the government ignored their advice,[1] they differed with it only on detail, not principle. Both presented the opinions of medical scientists as 'the science' – the only response to the pandemic based on knowledge.

But the fight against a public health threat is never only (and often not mainly) about access to medical science. If it was, South Africa would boast the lowest case and death numbers in Africa because it has more medical scientists and medical technology than other countries on the continent. But its case numbers and deaths are, in reality, the highest on the continent. Protecting public health is inevitably a social and political activity because it is, to a large degree, about how people behave; its goal is to encourage or force people to act in ways most likely to keep them alive and healthy. Medical science hopes to tell us how a health threat operates and what can be done to avoid it or to treat it. It cannot tell us how to ensure that people do what is required, whether those people are government ministers, those who wield private power over providing health care, or the citizenry.

To take but one example, which moved onto the agenda towards the end of 2020, medical science can develop a vaccine but decisions by political and economic power holders determine who enjoys access to it and politics may determine who is willing to take it. This point takes on greater urgency when there is no vaccine (for the vast majority of people) or cure and the only way to contain the virus is to prevent people spreading it. The role of government is essential and so is the relationship between government and citizens, whether this rests on mutual trust or the effective use of power by those in authority. Medical science helps keep the citizenry healthy but an approach which sees public health as a purely medical problem is certain to hide more than it reveals.

This reality was never recognised by the South African government. It did not appoint any social scientists to its Ministerial Advisory Committee (MAC), a choice which was criticised publicly in an editorial in the *South African Medical Journal* written by a researcher based at the Centre for the Aids Programme of Research in South Africa (CAPRISA) at the University of KwaZulu-Natal. Professor Salim Abdool Karim, who was chair of the MAC in 2020, is the long-time director of CAPRISA.[2] Later that year, in June, the then minister of health, Dr Zweli Mkhize, appointed a social and behavioural change committee, but again no social scientists were selected – the committee consisted of clergy and interest groups whose support the government felt it needed.[3] 'Following the science' clearly did not mean taking seriously anyone who studies society. Since one of the weaknesses in the country's approach was a failure to understand the realities experienced by people living in poverty, this may have ensured that the government's approach was not as guided by science as it claimed.

Nor does it necessarily require knowledge of medical science to analyse public health programmes. Many of the claims which medical scientists make about pandemics are based on interpretations of data which are available to anyone who keeps up with the daily news. Karim's response to Covid-19 was based on his claim that no country had avoided a severe epidemic. This makes a statement which can be understood – and challenged – by anyone who follows the news. The claim that those of us who challenge the opinions of scientists must be dismissed out of hand because we are amateurs claiming to be epidemiologists is an attempt to silence debate. No medical training is required to discover how many people in particular countries have tested positive for a disease and how many are officially reported to have died of it.

Scientific training is also not required to work out that scientists are, like judges who are also sometimes assumed to be infallible, human beings who have biases and prejudices like all other humans and that this might have as much to do with what they say about public health issues as with their scientific training. Precisely because public health is political, scientific opinions – and disagreements between scientists – are not principally a neutral report of, and debate on, the findings of experiments. It is impossible to say anything about public health without making assumptions about society, how it works and how it should work. And, since the way we view the world is often a product of our place in society, there is no reason why middle-class scientists should not share the prejudices of other middle-class people. Great harm may be done to society when we who have no medical training accept what scientists say without challenge when it seems to have more to do with their view of the world than their training or the research they undertake. It does not require training in medical science to detect scientists' biases and to point out how these influence their opinions.

This is why this book assumes that the fight against Covid-19 can be best understood through political analysis. This may sound like the rejection of medical science which prompted some to deny the reality of HIV and Aids or which, currently, wishes away Covid-19 and the measures used to fight it, including vaccines. It is not. Medical science plays an important role in the fight against pandemics. When HIV became a key concern in South Africa, ignoring or rejecting scientific findings cost hundreds of thousands of lives – in Brazil and parts of the United States, the same response to Covid-19 has had the same effect.

But, while medical science is indispensable in the fight against pandemics, success or failure depends on political decision-making. The core question raised by any society's response to a threat to public health is not whether it 'followed the science'. Nor is it whether it prevented the health system from being overwhelmed. It is whether it ensured that as few people as possible fell ill and as few as possible lost their lives. This, in turn, is a product of who decides how and whether to fight the epidemic, on what criteria, and how able they are to translate intentions into action. These decisions and abilities to implement them are the products of politics and so it is a study of the politics of how countries – or those who wield power within them – responded to the virus which allows us to understand and assess how effectively they coped with (and are coping with) Covid-19. Since responses to pandemics rely on human behaviour, the nature of particular societies and the relationship between the authorities and those they govern is also crucial. How countries respond to pandemics tells us much about them.

The phrase 'following the science' can also deflect political responsibility and so obstruct accountability. If governments are simply doing what scientists tell them to do, they cannot be blamed if what they do fails to prevent illness and death – or if the measures they adopt are resented by citizens. Many governments, including South Africa's, which claim to 'follow the science' don't always do this. But even when they do – and it has already been noted that, despite scientists' complaints, South Africa's government response was broadly consistent with the view of scientists – this hides the reality that, where the science is unclear and scientists offer differing views, 'following the science' is a political choice which makes some science more congenial to governments than others. The central argument of this book is that the advice of the scientists and the response of the government were products not of technical knowledge but of (unstated) political and social views which are products of the way South African society works and the attitudes this instils in people. By opening discussion on this question, the book hopes to contribute to ensuring that future responses to health threats follow a path which results in fewer people falling ill and fewer dying.

This book seeks to make sense of South Africa's response to Covid-19: it argues that the country did not do well because its elites, which include the participants in its public debate, see Western Europe and North America as the centre of the universe – the focal point to which the country is compared, even when the purpose is to show that South Africa is doing better in some respects than its richer objects of attention. It will try to show that this in turn is a product of the country's internal division into two 'worlds', one of which resembles the global North while the other is much like the rest of the global

South. An obvious implication is that if this is why the country did not contain Covid-19, it is also partly why it battles to overcome its other social and economic challenges.

I am grateful to Wits University Press for enabling me to write the book and the Humanities Faculty at the University of Johannesburg, which continues to offer me an academic home, encouragement and the means to contribute to scholarly and public debate on how we might build a South African democracy which includes and values all who live within its borders. While this book examines the country's response to a medical emergency, it is a further contribution to this vital debate.

LIST OF ACRONYMS

Africa CDC	Africa Centres for Disease Control and Prevention
ANC	African National Congress
BBC	British Broadcasting Corporation
BRICS	Brazil, Russia, India, China, South Africa
CAPRISA	Centre for the Aids Programme of Research in South Africa
DA	Democratic Alliance
GCRO	Gauteng City-Region Observatory
HSRC	Human Sciences Research Council
MAC	Ministerial Advisory Committee
NCCC	National Coronavirus Command Council
NICD	National Institute for Communicable Diseases
SAHPRA	South African Health Products Regulatory Authority
SAIRR	South African Institute of Race Relations
SAMRC	South African Medical Research Council
TB	tuberculosis
USA	United States of America
WHO	World Health Organization

INTRODUCTION

South Africa is in Africa but, if its response to Covid-19 is a guide, not of it.

Strangely, for a country whose public debate is usually loud and polarised, there was little discussion in 2020 of how well the country fared in combatting the virus. In the mainstream, it was simply assumed that it did well, despite over three-quarters of a million cases and over 20 000 deaths by late November. This was followed by a more severe 'second wave' which proved at least twice as deadly as the first. None of this caused alarm in the public debate. It was, throughout the year, common to encounter people who insisted that South Africa was 'doing well' in limiting Covid-19's effect.

But on what was this claim based? We were never told. Since South Africa's case numbers were at one stage fifth highest in the world and, by the end of November, still in the top 15 although it is only the planet's twenty-fifth biggest country,[1] the self-congratulation seems unjustified. It certainly did not 'do well' compared to the countries of East Asia, most of whose case and death figures were a fraction of this country's (or New Zealand, which appears to have largely defeated Covid-19). It did not 'do well' compared to the rest of the African continent. For a long while, it experienced as many cases and deaths as the rest of the continent combined. While its share of both dropped towards the end of the year, it was still, by a large distance, the African country with the most cases and loss of life. But this made no impact on the South African debate. The virus's impact on Africa was rarely reported on by the media and the comparison between South Africa's experience and that of the rest of the continent was ignored by the debate.

The rest of Africa would seem to be the most obvious area to which South Africa should be compared. Covid-19 cases and deaths may not simply be a consequence of how well governments have done in combatting the virus. Climate might matter since the virus is airborne and spreads more rapidly indoors (and so also in countries where climate forces people inside). Age profile might also affect figures because young people were, during 2020, less likely to suffer severe illness or to die of the virus. So might the living conditions of most people. It could be argued that the states of East Asia (and Australasia) are very different to South Africa and that its experience cannot be compared to theirs. But it is hard to make this argument about the rest of Africa, the part of the world to which South Africa's climate, age profile and living conditions (for the majority) are closest. It has no in-built disadvantages compared to the rest of the continent and should therefore experience case numbers and fatality rates similar to those of the rest of Africa (or better, given its more sophisticated health-care facilities). The fact that it was far more affected than any other African country must mean that it did not do well at all.

The only reason for not measuring South Africa against the rest of the continent is a deep-rooted bias. The debate disregards how Africa has dealt with Covid-19 because it ignores it on all other issues too. About the only time the rest of the continent features in South Africa's debates is when it is dragged in to settle arguments which are about something else. On one side of the fence, the continent may be cited as a cautionary tale ('if we carry on like this we will be as bad as the rest of Africa'). On the other, people and institutions which are insensitive to the concerns of black South Africans will be accused of contempt for Africa. In both cases, Africa is an idea, not a place, still less one peopled with complicated human beings. For the rest, the continent is largely ignored. News from the rest of Africa rarely makes headlines and some international news outlets give more prominence than South Africa's media to African developments. Nor is there evidence that the media's indifference to Africa deprives South Africans of news and insights they want. The rest of the continent evokes little interest in citizens who engage on digital media (more commonly called 'social' media despite the fact that they are owned by large profit-making corporations) or as consumers of traditional news. The media reflect the lack of interest; they do not create it.

Despite the vagueness of the claim, it is not difficult to work out in comparison to whom South Africa is assumed to have done well. Brazil has done poorly, but the South African debate does not think or talk about Brazil. During 2021, India, after initially containing the virus, experienced a horrifying 'second wave' (if cases and deaths are calculated as a percentage of population, its figures were not much different from South Africa's but years of underfunding ensured that its health facilities could not cope).[2] But the debate does not think or talk of India – its ordeal was noticed only because it was covered in detail by Western media. When South Africa's government ministers and scientists talk of 'the world', they mean Western Europe and North America (the United States and Canada). Sometimes this is explicit – it was common for South Africa's scientists to compare its experience directly to that of Western Europe or the USA.[3] But it is also implied. Not long after Covid-19 arrived in South Africa, Karim, who as chair of the MAC on Covid-19 was, in effect, the government's chief scientific advisor, declared that a severe epidemic was inevitable because no country had avoided one.[4] Since at the time (April 2020) many countries, including the entire African continent, had done precisely that,

3

his remark made no sense unless what he really meant to say is that no country of interest to the South African elite had avoided one, which meant no major Western European or North American country.

The assumption that 'the world' is, in reality, the countries of the 'West' is deeply ingrained in South Africa, despite frequent ritual salutes to 'Africa' or the countries of the BRICS alliance, Brazil, Russia, India and China. It shapes not only the debate, but thinking on public policy. It is a consequence both of the country's history, particularly its specific form of minority rule, and of its current reality, marked by the existence of two very different worlds in one country. Inevitably, this reality framed its official response to Covid-19, ensuring that the country with the most sophisticated health facilities on the continent was, by a considerable margin, more severely affected than anywhere else in Africa.

It is, of course, necessary to justify this core assumption that South Africa did not 'do well' by comparing its experience in greater detail with that of the rest of Africa. An obvious danger of writing about Covid-19 while the pandemic is still in progress is that events move very quickly. At the time this book was being written, South Africa had passed through a 'second wave' of increased infections which the rest of the continent was also experiencing. While this book discusses the 'second wave' when this is necessary to help understand the issues it explores, its chief focus is on developments until the end of November 2020.

This is necessary because the virus has not disappeared and the details of case and fatality numbers change every day. The discovery of vaccines has added a new dynamic and it is too early for a full assessment. A line must be drawn somewhere and the obvious place to draw it is at the end of the first phase of the virus, which is over and so more easily analysed. More important, the 'second wave' – if that is indeed what it is, for there is good reason to challenge the claim that what happened in December 2020, as case numbers grew sharply in several provinces, was very different from what had come before – has not altered the arguments made in this book; on the contrary, it has confirmed them. The pattern created in much of 2020 has persisted into 2021 and, although the rest of Africa experienced higher case and death numbers, by the end of February 2021, South Africa's epidemic was still substantially more severe as a proportion of population than that of any other country on the continent. Events in late 2020 and early 2021 add nuance to the analysis offered here but do not challenge it.

SOUTH AFRICA AND AFRICA

Official numbers of cases and deaths in South Africa and the rest of Africa between the onset of the virus and the end of November 2020 starkly underline Covid-19's vastly disproportionate impact on one country.

By 30 November, South Africa had recorded 787 702 cases and 21 477 deaths of people who had tested positive.[5] The official figures also insist on recording recoveries, which, on that date, stood at 730 633, giving a recovery rate of 93 per cent. This recovery figure is dutifully reported in news media and seems designed to signal that, despite the high numbers, the country is indeed doing well since over nine in ten people who test positive recover. But this implied self-congratulation is misleading. Calculations using World Health Organization (WHO) figures show that the global case fatality rate for Covid-19 – the percentage of infected people who lose their lives – was 2.3 per cent on 30 November. The highest case fatality rate was Mexico's at 9.5 per cent.[6] So, on average, 97.7 per cent of people who are infected recover and, at worst, nine in ten do. A recovery rate of 93 per cent reflects how Covid-19 affects humans, not how well a country is dealing with it. Yet it is implicitly presented as a sign that the country is doing well at ensuring that those who contract Covid-19 recover. Also, the recovery figures reflect the number of people who tested positive and then tested negative. They say nothing about the fact that some infected people endure 'long Covid', which means that they experience symptoms indefinitely after testing negative.[7] Not all those listed as recovered are now healthy.

In July, at the (then) peak of its epidemic, South Africa had the fifth highest number of cases on the planet, behind only the USA, Brazil, Russia and India.[8] By end November, it had dropped to sixteenth but this does not take population into account.[9] If cases and deaths are calculated as a percentage of population, South Africa had, during that period, double the cases and three times the deaths of India – it also experienced more deaths, although not cases, than Russia. It had also detected about the same number of cases (although significantly fewer deaths) as Iran, which is viewed as a country which has been hit particularly hard, and more cases (but again far fewer deaths) than Mexico, which is seen in the same light.[10] According to official figures, the only countries in comparison to which South Africa can be said to have done well are some in Latin America – and the USA and Europe. (India's 'second wave' in 2021 was also more severe although, if population is taken into account, the number of cases and deaths in India was not hugely different to those in South Africa's 'second wave', even if the scale of devastation was greater.)

Comparison with the rest of the continent further undermines the claim that South Africa did well. The reality noted earlier – that, up to November, the country reported about as many cases and fatalities as all other African countries combined – held steady for months. Roughly the same number of illnesses and deaths as 53 other countries combined is not a triumph. During November, it was reported that, according to the African Centres for Disease Control and Prevention (Africa CDC), African cases had reached two million;[11] South Africa's share of cases had reduced to around 40 per cent of the total while deaths were just under 50 per cent. There seems, however, to be some doubt about the figures since the WHO's Covid-19 dashboard reported some 1.5 million confirmed cases in Africa and 33 710 deaths,[12] which would make South Africa's share of cases 53 per cent and of deaths 63 per cent. But even if the figures which reduce South Africa's share of cases and deaths to around four in ten are accurate, South Africans comprise less than five per cent of Africa's population. By the South African government's own reckoning, the contrast between its experience and that of its neighbours is even starker. In a presentation to the WHO in late August 2020, the minister of health, Zweli Mkhize, revealed that, within the Southern African Development Community (SADC) region, South Africa was responsible for 90 per cent of cases and 91 per cent of deaths[13] despite making up only a little more than 20 per cent of the population.[14]

South Africa stood out in another way too – women bore the brunt of cases and deaths, a reality different from that in other African countries which record the gender of people who test positive for Covid 19 (most don't do this). According to Mkhize's presentation, women comprised 58 per cent of Covid-19 cases.[15] He did not give fatality figures for men and women but a study by the African Population Health Research Centre, based in Kenya, found that 49 per cent of South Africans who died of the disease were women. By contrast, in the other African countries which kept these records, women account for 40 per cent of cases and 30 per cent of deaths.[16] A Gauteng City-Region Observatory (GCRO) team found that: 'This gender gap is largely occurring for women of working age (from 20 to 65 years of age) and for the very elderly.' Although 'quite a few countries in the developed world' reported female cases above 55 per cent, 'the key difference is that in those countries the majority of this gender bias is explained by cases among those over 80 years of age'.[17] So South Africa's women are worst affected but not mainly because they live longer and so are more likely to be at an age where they are at risk.

In a separate article, the GCRO research team noted that, according to the National Income Dynamics Study-Coronavirus Rapid Mobile

Survey (NIDS-CRAM), which researches the social and economic impact of the pandemic, women accounted for two-thirds of the net job losses in the initial months of the epidemic. Women were more likely than men to live in households that reported running out of money for food in April 2020 and more women than men were 'living with children and spending more hours on childcare since the start of the lockdown'. They added that research data show that women were more likely to be infected because they are more exposed to risk factors: crowded conditions, relying on public transport, 'poor health status' and 'living in households with pre-existing conditions'. Women are also less likely to have access to medical aid and 'are more likely to rely on public health care services'.[18]

Comparing a country with a continent or a region may be a little abstract. We can bring home the point more clearly by comparing South Africa's cases and deaths with those of some other African countries. The second worst affected during 2020 was Egypt – by late November it had reported some 116 000 cases and 6 650 deaths.[19] If we bear in mind that South Africa's population is around 59 million and Egypt's 102 million,[20] then South Africa experienced ten times more cases and six times as many deaths. The worst affected sub-Saharan country was Nigeria, which reported 67 557 cases and 1 173 deaths.[21] This is about one-twelfth the number of South African cases and almost one-twentieth of its deaths. Since Nigeria's population is 206 million,[22] it had, as a proportion of population, around 2 per cent of South Africa's cases and 1.5 per cent of its deaths. Eight months after the virus began spreading in Africa, South Africa's recorded case numbers and fatalities vastly exceeded those of every other country on the continent.

South Africans who are aware of this reality usually insist that the vast gap between the country's record and that of the rest of the continent can be easily explained: the other countries do not test as many of their citizens and their death statistics are unreliable, so it can safely be assumed that their case and death numbers are much higher than the official figures indicate. It is true that other African countries do not test as much as South Africa – Africa CDC acknowledges this.[23] So, it can be safely assumed that the official figures on African cases are underestimates. But then so are those in every other country – medical scientists acknowledge that some cases are never counted in an epidemic.[24] The question is whether African states' data collection limitations mean that so many cases and deaths are not being reported that the claim that South Africa has not performed well in comparison to the rest of the continent may be false. This is highly unlikely. People tend to notice when those around them fall ill, let alone when they lose loved ones. Only in societies in which all the world's media are effectively silenced would authorities have a chance of covering up many deaths and no African countries fit that description.

When Covid-19 began to spread around the world, it was frequently predicted that it would devastate Africa. When it didn't, media in the global North (or those who noticed) used this reality to further stigmatise Africans. One report quoted Professor Shabir Madhi, a Wits University vaccinologist who is interviewed more often by the media than Karim, speculating that 'poor conditions' might protect Africans from the disease, apparently because they may have contracted diseases which enabled them to build an immunity.[25] (This view was reported deferentially despite its failure to explain why people living in poverty in Latin America and the United States were severely affected.) He did not claim that large numbers of cases and deaths were not recorded.[26]

The British Broadcasting Corporation (BBC), in its continuing zeal to demonstrate that Africa is indeed conforming to its stereotype, claims to have found evidence that people were buried in Somalia, with their deaths not reflecting in official figures.[27] But this appears to be the only report to make this claim – it seems likely that, if Somalis were indeed dying in much greater numbers than the official figures claim, other reports would have followed, just as it seems equally likely that, if this was a widespread reality in Africa, we would have read or heard more accounts of this sort. South African medical scientists who share mainstream biases about Africa's capacity, accept that there is no great cover up and that lack of testing is not the explanation. Karim, in an interview with *Nature*, noted: 'Some people say it's because those countries don't test enough. But even if you don't test, you still will see an increase of hospital admissions and deaths. So that's not the real reason.'[28] Madhi's reaction, noted above, also appears to accept that case numbers are significantly lower than expected. To amplify the point, the tech billionaire Bill Gates – who, with his then wife Melinda, runs a foundation which devotes attention to medical programmes in Africa – declared in the last days of 2020 that he 'does not understand why coronavirus numbers have not been as high as predicted in Africa'. The Gateses had predicted widespread carnage in Africa as the virus ripped through populations. He said he was glad that they were wrong but, consistent with his admission that he had no explanation, did not offer one.[29]

The implied claim that the virus is decimating the continent but that this is being hidden by incompetence or deceit is not surprising: Africa is routinely stigmatised as the epicentre of incompetence and incapacity. The view that it cannot possibly be doing well in its response to Covid-19 has been assiduously advanced by the BBC, whose reporting seems heavily influenced by a desire to show that Africa can't possibly be doing better than the 'civilised' countries of Western Europe. It declared that: 'It's also worth pointing out that for some African countries, it is impossible to know what exactly is happening due to a lack of any data or data being incomplete.'[30] In 2021, a new twist – insisting that Africa was already engulfed by unreported illnesses and deaths, or was about to be – became a theme of campaigners who wanted rich countries to share vaccines. Sweeping claims were made, often on the strength of anecdotal evidence or none at all, to bolster the case for strong action to inoculate the continent.[31] But the evidence then offered a different picture.

African countries' response to the virus has been coordinated by Africa CDC, created by the African Union. Africa CDC works with a variety of partners, notably the WHO, whose African region has also played a significant role in attempts to contain Covid-19 (including, according to South Africa's government, this country's). Its head, Dr John Nkengasong, says that 'even with limited data', African health officials are 'increasingly sure that most coronavirus cases are asymptomatic – he puts the figure at 70–80% – and that deaths are relatively low'. He adds: 'our deaths ... are not as high as in other parts of the world' – 'member states are looking actively as to whether deaths are occurring massively in the community, and that is not the case'.[32]

The consensus view among African health officials that up to four out of five cases are not identified because the infected person is asymptomatic and so does not present for testing does not suggest a desire to uncover unpalatable evidence. This strengthens the credibility of their findings on deaths – that large numbers are not being covered up or simply ignored. Unlike much of the South African debate, Africa CDC sees South Africa as an African country and so the comments on asymptomatic cases and on deaths refer to this country too. While we can assume that cases and deaths are under-reported in the rest of Africa, we can assume this in South Africa (and everywhere else) too – in September, Mkhize said that 12 million people, one-fifth of the population, may have been affected.[33] It is also important to note that, when the 'second wave' began in Africa, this was reflected in rising case numbers and deaths which were reported by African countries and by Africa CDC.[34] If Africa's medical scientists had both the capacity and the will to notice and report increases in cases and fatalities, it seems reasonable to assume that they did not miss or conceal a severe 'first wave'.

Why many African states managed, during 2020, to reduce cases and deaths is discussed in chapter 2. But the evidence presented here shows that South Africa has been much more severely affected than the rest of the continent. The book will show that this was not despite the fact that it has a more sophisticated health system than any other African country but because of it – or at least because of the realities which ensured that the country had seeming advantages which others lacked.

CHAPTER

1

One Country, Two Realities

Since it became a democracy in 1994, South Africa has been, in law, one united country. The apartheid system's attempt to justify white domination by forcing black people to become citizens of legally independent statelets is over. But, while it has one common citizenship, it houses two worlds. This has shaped its fight against Covid-19.

It is common to point out that, according to official data, South Africa is the most unequal country in the world.[1] It is equally common to remark on the contrast between the privileges and luxuries a minority enjoys and the poverty and squalor in which most are forced to live. So much of a commonplace is it that, in 2019, ahead of that year's elections, *Time* magazine devoted its cover story to pointing out precisely this.[2] But that hardly makes the country unique: inequality has been growing across the globe for decades[3] and it is hardly the only African country in which there are large disparities between the lives of the well-off and those of the poor – and where some live in comfortable suburbs, many others in underserviced slums. What makes

South Africa a standout in Africa is that the divide is less one between rich and poor as between inhabitants of two very different worlds. This makes the country more similar to those in Latin America and so it may be no coincidence that Latin America, too, has experienced high levels of Covid-19 cases and deaths.[4]

To understand why this is so, we need to remind ourselves of the country's history. Under colonialism and apartheid, the two worlds were a product of law enforced by an army and police force. Initially a Dutch and then a British colony, the country formally became a Republic in 1960. But the attitudes and habits which underpinned colonisation survived. This was hardly surprising since so too did white rule, which sought to transplant the dominant culture of Europe and North America (or, since in those countries, as elsewhere, culture is diverse and ever-changing, what white South Africans believed that culture to be) on African soil. Most English-speaking whites looked to Britain as a model, often comparing its 'civilisation' with the supposed roughness and crudity of white Afrikaans speakers.[5] And, while many of these English speakers are not liberals, the political philosopher Richard Turner's remark that white liberals under apartheid '… believe that "western civilisation" is adequate, and superior to other forms, but also that blacks can, through education, attain [its] level'[6] applies more broadly to English-speaking South Africa. Most Afrikaans speakers – those who supported the system – were more likely to see Germany or the Netherlands as a model. They also had a more complicated reaction, chiding 'the West' for not understanding the need for apartheid. But the fact that they cared about what the West thought revealed the truth: that they too craved the approval of 'civilised' Western countries. In the early 1950s, Piet Meyer, a key Afrikaner Nationalist ideologue, told Western intellectuals that 'the Afrikaner nation' was a 'young West European nation'.[7]

These attitudes were given form in apartheid society. White areas, lifestyles and institutions essentially implanted Western Europe and the

Unites States on African soil: visitors would remark that the suburbs of the major cities resembled Southern California. Like the citizens of those societies, whites enjoyed the vote and civil liberties – provided that they did not identify overly with black demands. Not only were black people excluded (except as labourers serving the needs of the whites who inhabited this world) by law, the division of the country into different worlds was government policy and ideology. Races and ethnic groups were held to possess a distinctive culture which would be fatally diluted if mixed with others and this was said to be a rationale for strict racial separation. Apartheid ideologues also extolled those among the colonised who, in their view, knew that they belonged to a different world and had no need to leave it. According to Daan de Wet Nel, then minister of bantu administration and development, 'The Zulu is proud to be a Zulu, the Xhosa is proud to be a Xhosa and the Venda is proud to be a Venda, just as proud as they were a hundred years ago.'[8] He meant that they knew their place and had no wish to join the white world of suburban homes, corporate office towers and malls.

This ideology began to erode as white Afrikaners became wealthier and more integrated into 'Western' society, and as apartheid proved increasingly unenforceable. By the time the system ended in 1994, some black people were already being admitted to this world, albeit in a subordinate position: they were allowed to perform skilled work, occupy some white-collar jobs and, from 1985, live in the cities whether or not their labour was needed by white employers. Cultural and sporting apartheid eroded so blacks were no longer excluded, at least legally, from competing with whites on the field and performing in front of them on the stage and screen. By the time apartheid formally ended, in 1994, it was discredited and not even right-wing white politicians or professionals would be caught echoing De Wet Nel's view that two worlds were ordained by nature.

But the two worlds did not end. The reasons have been analysed elsewhere[9] but the outline must be sketched here because it is the key to understanding the country's response to Covid-19. In essence, the core goal of government (supported by implication by many of society's influential voices and interests) since 1994 has been to extend to everyone what whites enjoyed under apartheid. The end of white rule did not, as might have been expected, produce a decisive move away from the divisions of the apartheid era towards a culture and institutions which met the needs of all citizens. One possible consequence of a social reality like that under apartheid – in which one group enjoys amenities, rights and privileges by dominating another – is that the way of life of the dominating group may come to be seen as the norm to which the society should aspire. That is largely what has happened in South Africa after apartheid.

It is easy to see why white citizens should want their world under apartheid to be the goal – it enables them to continue to live much as they had lived before. But the new black leadership shared this view. Whites lived well under apartheid and the new governing elite believed that black people should not be expected to make do with less than their dominators enjoyed. If the new elite did what logic suggested it needed to do – insist that everyone, including apartheid's beneficiaries, would need to make do with less than what a tenth of the population had enjoyed by dominating the rest – it would reinforce white prejudices which assume that government by black people always ends in a reduction of 'standards'. Particularly when the government was led by President Thabo Mbeki (formally for nine years but, since Nelson Mandela adopted a deliberate strategy of leaving much of the running of the government to Mbeki to show that a smooth transition to competent leadership was possible, in reality 12 to 14 years), the core goal was to show whites, at home and abroad, that rule by black people could maintain the standards which whites were assumed to expect. The government's priority was thus those tasks which whites were thought to value.[10]

The politicians, officials, academics and journalists who adopted this approach would be shocked and angry if they were told they were preserving the divisions of the past in a new shell, but this was exactly what they were doing. Precisely because it was impossible to extend to everyone what only a few had enjoyed because they controlled the means of force and used it to exclude everyone else, the approach retained the division between insiders and outsiders which was central to apartheid. The development path since 1994 has centred on squeezing as many black people as possible into the institutions of suburban society (including the upper reaches of the economy) rather than fundamentally changing them. Efforts to undo the inequities of apartheid have centred not on collapsing the divisions between insiders and outsiders but on trying to ensure that as many black people as possible become insiders. Despite many claims to the contrary, attempts to deracialise the economy have centred far less on providing black people with the resources and opportunities they need to build their own economic muscle than on pressing existing corporates to concede a greater black role.[11] Universities deracialised by expecting black students and faculty to adapt to the way they had always operated,[12] a pattern which sparked the Rhodes Must Fall student protests of 2015.[13]

It is this path which has ensured that South Africa, once divided into insiders and outsiders by law and by race, continues the divide without the obvious racial barriers which underpinned apartheid. Some of the symptoms are common to all countries, including many in Africa: income inequalities, high levels of unemployment and affluence for a few, poverty for most. But in other African countries, those who benefit from these arrangements are a small fraction of the population – in South Africa, the insiders could be up to a third of the citizenry. Nor do the elites in the other countries inherit institutions and patterns of behaviour built up over centuries of white settlement. In most, the colonisers were a small group of officials, soldiers and police and their families who returned to Europe when independence came. In those countries where colonisers settled – South Africa's neighbours Zimbabwe and Namibia, and also Kenya and Algeria – the white group was small or shrank on independence when almost all the colonisers left. In South Africa, despite high levels of white emigration, and constant white angst that their numbers are shrinking fast, some 4.6 million white people still lived in the country in mid-2019.[14]

In itself, this last statistic is of no great interest to anyone who does not believe that a country's racial composition gives it advantages or disadvantages. But, in contrast to the rest of the continent, millions of people remain in South Africa who see North America and Western Europe as the most important regions on the planet. If we add to this that the country's goal since 1994 has been to ensure that as many black people as possible are absorbed into the life world of this sizeable minority, the stratum of society which benefits from the formal economy has grown and is now no longer white only. Whether black people are inside or outside this world depends on whether they are able to participate in the formal economy: people who receive a wage and a salary are, to varying degrees, participants in the institutions and activities which white rule created. Some 9.6 million people were employed in September 2020, so the insider group is at least this large.[15] It is, in fact, significantly larger since the dependents of working people as well as retired people receiving private pensions and their immediate dependents[16] are also insiders since they benefit from the regular income which participation in the formal economy offers.

This does not mean that all the insiders enjoy similar incomes and lifestyles – the insider group ranges from unionised office cleaners to corporate chief executives. But it does mean that South Africa is the only country in Africa in which at least one-sixth of the society – 10 million out of a population of 59 million – and probably up to a third if immediate dependents are included, is 'locked into' the formal economy, a product of the Western-focused world which white rule brought and which majority rule has not sought to overturn. To varying degrees, this also means incorporation in a world which looks very much like that of the 'First World' – of which the affluent West is a crucial component.

At the lower end of the scale, insiders, defined as people who earn a wage or salary or other income from the formal economy (such as dividends and pensions), may live in crowded township houses or shacks, lack services, rely for news and entertainment on vernacular radio or the television channels offered by the national public broadcaster and enjoy limited access to the health and education systems. The outsiders live in a similar world, although for obvious reasons their homes are likely to be even more crowded (and more likely to be shacks) and they enjoy even less access to health care and schooling. If they happen to be women, they are likely to live in even poorer conditions than male outsiders and more likely to contract Covid-19 and to die from it. But a significant section of the insider group will own their homes and devices which enable them to connect with the world and each other in cyberspace; rely for their news and views on the internet, digital media and, for the more old fashioned, satellite television; belong to a medical aid scheme which grants them access to private care, offered in practices and hospitals which are much the same as those in the West; and send their children to suburban schools and then to university. The lives and experiences of outsiders follow a very different path.

This divide inevitably affects the way people see the world. The political commentator Aubrey Matshiqi has observed that, in South Africa's democracy, 'the political majority remain a cultural minority'.[17] The comment is often assumed to mean that white people, a political minority, determine what is culturally acceptable. This was part of what he meant, but not all of it. Another aspect of this reality is that the values and assumptions which govern mainstream social and political life are also those of a minority, to which the majority is expected to conform if they want to be taken seriously. A key element of this reality is that, in the insider world, Europe and North America are the centres of gravity.

It is important to clarify what this means. The insiders are divided by race and political perspective – some admire 'the West', others loudly reject it. But both see it as a focus. In public discussion of politics, the United States of America is discussed heatedly. So, albeit to a lesser extent, is Western Europe. Other regions might get a passing mention to make a point but there are few discussions of the Modi government in India or the Bolsonaro presidency in Brazil, despite the fact that both are South Africa's partners in the BRICS alliance (and, latterly, even when their Covid-19 cases and deaths have been widely covered by Western media). China might be mentioned as a problem or solution but its internal politics and the dynamics of its society are ignored. Events in Africa are barely discussed – when they are, the discussion is superficial and usually designed to make a point about domestic politics. Predictably, the same pattern is evident in academic or policy debates. It is very rare to see other African countries as useful models for policies and practices – it is far more common to look to Europe, North America or Australia. This is generally so whatever the race or political allegiance of the participants. During constitutional negotiations in the early 1990s, all the parties showed intense interest in German and Canadian federalism, none at all in that in Nigeria or India.[18] Discussions of negotiated economic compromises focus on Sweden, Germany or Ireland – never Mauritius, whose economic development depended heavily on economic bargaining.[19]

Since the insiders associate their life world with sophistication and modernity, black people who have not been incorporated into the world of the suburbs are a source of embarrassment, a sign that the society has not yet managed to elevate all its citizens to the status of suburban residents. But the shame is often not directed at the fact that the society has forced people to live in poverty. It is the people who live in poverty who are the embarrassment because they have not attained the 'standards' of the minority. One example is a debate on jobs which is underpinned by the belief that the country can and should extend to all the condition of most white people under apartheid, who were virtually assured a job in a shop, office or factory. These jobs are labelled 'decent' by the governing party (and many others),[20] which implies that earning a livelihood informally is 'indecent'. It is repeatedly claimed that social grants create 'dependency',[21] which can be avoided only by acquiring a job. Both views ignore the reality that formal jobs are under pressure everywhere and there is no realistic prospect of offering each adult a job in the foreseeable future. The dismissal of grants fails to see that they are the only feasible route to sustaining most South Africans under current circumstances and are often used to stimulate local economies and open new avenues to productive work.[22] The assumption that white life patterns under apartheid are the desired end point of an appropriate development path keeps alive a mythology which sees the people of the townships and shack settlements as a deficiency.

The South African divide runs deeper than a difference between those who have and those who lack. History has ensured that it is the only country in Africa where two very different social and economic worlds cohabit. The suburbs – understood as a symbol of the insider life described here – inhabit a different world to the outsiders in townships and shacks. And the divide between them mirrors the international contrast between the 'First' and the 'Third' worlds. The 'First', as we know, is associated with prosperity, sophistication and competence, the 'Third' with poverty, ignorance, incompetence and incapacity. The distinction between them is crude – it also expresses deep-rooted prejudices about the superiority of some lifestyles and cultures over others. Features associated with the 'First World' are found in societies labelled 'Third World' and vice versa. But it captures an important South African reality – that a section of the society lives in circumstances much like those in the wealthy Western countries and, equally important, sees the world much as mainstream inhabitants of those countries do, while the majority live very different lives, encounter very different experiences and have different priorities. The divide is indeed one between two worlds which are based on different assumptions and in which what is a priority and what is not differs markedly.

Only one of the two worlds enjoys influence in South Africa's official understanding of itself. Politics and policy debate is the terrain of the insiders, for all politics is insider politics: the outsiders lack the resources or the power to influence a debate in which they are always talked about but never heard. Discussion of how the country should address its challenges is inevitably phrased in the language of the insiders and reflects their priorities and concerns (the social grants disparaged by many insiders are so important to outsiders that they largely shape their voting choices).[23] Their priorities set the boundaries of what may be taken seriously and what is dismissed as irrelevant. Since insider status is a consequence of participation in the market economy, it follows that, among this section of society, the expression of particular interests is especially important. Insiders are able to combine in associations far more easily than outsiders – the organisations they form, precisely because their members are insiders, are able to make themselves heard, not least because they can often rely on the media to report what they say. This power further strengthens the pattern in which insider voices monopolise the policy debate.

The divide between insiders and outsiders can ensure that important social campaigns are exercises in collective blindness even as they shine a light on realities which need urgent attention. During much of 2020, as Covid-19 spread, the government focused attention on 'gender-based violence', a peculiarly technical term for the often-lethal violence directed at South Africa's women. The campaign was necessary, but it addressed only part of the problem. For, while women were undoubtedly dying at the hands of violent men, they were also, as the Introduction showed, dying of the virus in numbers higher than those in the rest of Africa – not because of some biological accident but because the insiders who rightly lamented the overt violence against them failed to notice that their deaths at the hands of Covid-19 were also a product of policies and practices which made their lives cheaper. While Ramaphosa labelled violence against women the country's 'second pandemic',[24] he did not even mention that far more women were dying of the first pandemic than in other African countries and that this was a consequence of how they were forced to live. Even in their moments of compassion, the insiders find it impossible to see into the lives of 'Third World' South Africa.

It is easy to caricature the differences between the two worlds. As mentioned earlier, many in the 'First World' are highly critical of the West's role in colonisation and apartheid. Because the governing party enjoys historic ties with countries which are perceived (not always accurately) to have helped it in the fight against apartheid, and because its post-1994 foreign policy has tended to judge other countries purely on the strength of what they are able to offer South Africa, it sometimes acts in ways which might seem to show that it not only sees beyond the West but can support its 'enemies' – by nominating Cuba's external medical programme for the Nobel Price, for example.[25] Many in the 'Third World' majority may well share some of the values of the 'First World' mainstream, not least because television and radio are underpinned by this view of the world.

Conflict within 'First World' South Africa is extremely common. A quarter century of democracy has not eliminated racial divisions. Whites continue to wield much of the economic power,[26] and black people have been incorporated into 'First World' South Africa on unequal terms. This ensures continued tension. And, while the government has become deeply embedded in this world, it is held in contempt by it. Corruption and government ineffectiveness give good reason for much of this anger. But it is also born of an assumption by whites that black-ruled countries always fail and a growing cultural divide between a black middle and affluent class which has embraced the 'First World' and a government whose roots in 'liberation' politics, a very different milieu to that of the marketplace and the suburb, make it seem to many black people who have made it into the marketplace as a model of the past from which they hope to escape. The 'First World' is convinced that it is governed by a 'Third World' government, ignoring the degree to which the government shares most of the attitudes and assumptions of the 'First World' and to which those who serve in it also enjoy its lifestyle.

But this does not alter the reality that South Africa's enduring past has bequeathed it two societies in one, and that one, which includes the political class, business and the professions and those in the media and the academy who shape the country's priorities, sees the world in ways which assume, often perhaps unconsciously, the centrality of Western Europe and North America. It assumes, too, that the majority outside their world needs to be told what is good for it because it dwells in ignorance and incapacity. Access to power and resources ensures that the 'First World' decides what is to be done and the majority is obliged to adapt.

It is these realities which shaped the country's response to Covid-19. The 'First World' politicians and scientists, their eyes fixed firmly on the West, and convinced that their section of the society was required to think and plan for an ignorant and incompetent majority, framed a response to Covid-19 which conformed to these biases. Soon, the associations and interest groups mentioned earlier, often supported by the scientists and always assured a platform in the media, reinforced this, insisting that the response to the virus give priority to their interests. The result was an approach which ensured an official case and death rate which greatly exceeded that of any other country in Africa.

CHAPTER

2

Following the Science

From the time the first cases of Covid-19 were identified in South Africa, the government insisted that it would 'follow the science'.[1] This was greeted with excitement by medical scientists and many who shape the public debate. Their response was understandable for two reasons: one was a product of international developments, the other the result of recent South African history.

The global trend is one in which (usually right-wing) governments and citizens deny the reality of Covid-19. They minimise its severity and reject measures to prevent its spread, ranging from face masks to restrictions on economic, social and religious activity. This response is often seen as 'anti-science'[2] because it denies available knowledge and is accompanied by claims which are supported by no credible evidence.[3] In the initial stages of the virus's spread, much of this reaction was prompted by opposition to protective measures, either because they harmed the economic interests of the 'anti-scientists' or because government measures which tell citizens that they may not gather in bars and restaurants or attend religious services were considered an interference in personal enjoyment or expression. (Later, when vaccines were developed, rejection of the science became more complicated, stretching from right-wing conspiracy theorists to black people who may be reacting to a history of abuse by medical science.[4])

Its effect was always to compromise health and lives. The two countries whose leaders were most identified with this approach, the United States of America and Brazil, suffered particularly severe outbreaks. While, as will be seen, this was a rejection of common sense as much as of science, it was widely perceived as an insistence on placing political and economic considerations ahead of hard scientific evidence which showed that the virus is potentially deadly and that swift and strong measures are needed to protect against it. When governments were urged to 'follow the science', this meant that they should place the health of their citizens ahead of other priorities. It was assumed that they could best do this by listening to scientists rather than right-wing ideologues.

The government's response to the arrival of Covid-19 seemed to indicate both that it took the virus seriously and that it planned to rely on scientific advice. On the first score, on 15 March 2020, ten days after the first case was reported, the government declared a national state of disaster which entitled it to take emergency measures and to restrict activity to deal with the pandemic.[5] This remained in force during 2020 and into 2021. It established the National Coronavirus Command Council (NCCC) chaired by the president and the minister of co-operative government and traditional affairs, Dr Nkosazana Dlamini Zuma, whose department was responsible for the state of disaster regulations. The NCCC consisted of most of the Cabinet – 20 of 33 members – representatives of a security structure comprising the army, police and intelligence services, and the directors general (the most senior civil servants) in all the government departments represented.[6] The NCCC decided the government's response to the virus.

On the second, as noted above, Mkhize appointed a MAC which Karim chaired and which appears to have included all medical scientists whose work could help it respond to the pandemic, and in June also established a social and behavioural change committee. In September, as scientists became more confident that vaccines would be developed to fight the virus, he established a specific MAC on vaccines which included scientists, government officials, regulators and a representative of Biovac, the South African public–private partnership meant to develop vaccine manufacture.[7] It relied on the work of modellers, particularly the South African Covid-19 Modelling Consortium which consisted of researchers from the universities of Cape Town, Stellenbosch and the Witwatersrand, and the official National Institute of Communicable Diseases (NICD), which produced 'the main model' that the government used.[8] The work of other teams of modellers was used to assist national and provincial governments to plan.[9] In addition, the government enjoyed access to the research of the South African Medical Research Council (SAMRC), an institution created by law, and the NICD, which serves the government and other southern African countries.

During the pandemic, the NCCC – whose military title did nothing to dispel suspicions that it was more interested in controlling citizens than supporting them – was accused by some scientists of not 'following the science'. But, at this initial stage, that lay in the future. The government appeared to be signalling that it was fully committed to the fight against the virus and that it planned to use scientific knowledge to do this.

The recent domestic history which ensured that this approach was welcomed by scientists, the media and some citizens was the government's response, in the first few years of the twenty-first century, to a previous epidemic, HIV and Aids. Its effect was greatly worsened by the response of then president Thabo Mbeki who was hostile to the scientific consensus on the virus and to the scientists who urged that it be applied in South Africa. Some critics believed that Mbeki treated the science with scorn because it required his government to distribute, at its expense, medicine to millions of people and that he believed this would make it difficult to balance the budget. Mbeki's own statements suggested that he reacted as he did because he feared that the mainstream view on HIV and Aids would be used by racial bigots to claim falsely that the disease was spread by the sexual habits of black people.[10] But whatever the reason, the only scientists to whom he gave a sympathetic hearing were a small group of dissidents whose claims were discredited by the mainstream. Activists campaigning for affordable treatment for people living with Aids made much of the 'marginalisation' of the scientists: Mbeki's attitude was compared to Lysenkoism – Joseph Stalin's embrace of the ideas of the pseudo-scientist Lysenko, whose theories he declared to be state doctrine, so forcing scientists with more credible opinions into silence.[11]

The Ramaphosa government's response to Covid-19 was the polar opposite to Mbeki's. Karim, its MAC chair, was one of the scientists whose work on HIV and Aids Mbeki rejected; the committee included others who had been relegated to the margins during Mbeki's tenure. It made much of its partnership with scientists, some of whom it afforded platforms to inform the country of current evidence on Covid-19. The government's response was led by the minister of health, Zweli Mkhize, a medical doctor who was a classmate of Karim's at medical school. Activists and journalists, as well as Karim himself, marvelled at the contrast between this response and Mbeki's stance on Aids.[12] Shortly after the virus reached the country, Ramaphosa underlined the government's enthusiasm for science by announcing that it would respond with a 'risk adjusted strategy' to Covid-19 which would enable it to impose restrictions when and where required.[13] He promised that the government would use extensive screening and testing to identify people who had contracted Covid-19.[14] The scientific (and technocratic) language contrasted sharply with Aids denialism and elicited much admiration for the government's respect for science. This time, it seemed, it was guided by knowledge, not politics. Some scientists became media celebrities as the country waited for them to guide it out of danger.

But the hope that this alliance between science and government would produce an effective response to Covid-19 brushed aside important realities. Chief among them was the very real difference between Aids and Covid-19. When Aids became contentious in South Africa (from the early 2000s to Mbeki's resignation in 2008), the science was clear: scientists knew how people became infected and what needed to be done when they were. Most importantly, treatments had been discovered, antiretroviral drugs, which allowed infected people to live long and normal lives. The demand that the government 'be guided by the science' boiled down to little more than the insistence that it make a serious effort to fight the epidemic, in particular by making life-saving medicine available to people who could not afford it. Much of the 'denialism' of Mbeki and his health minister, Dr Manto Tshabalala-Msimang, was motivated by a refusal to do that.[15] Both sides knew what the mainstream science was – they could not agree on whether to follow it.

Covid-19 is a new illness and the science is evolving. To name but one of many examples, in the early stages of the pandemic it was assumed that only droplets on surfaces spread the infection. Later, evidence showed that it was airborne, which required different preventive strategies.[16] Much of what was passed off as 'state of the art' science in the early days of the pandemic – distancing, washing hands and not touching faces – was not the result of research on Covid-19: they were standard public health measures which had been used to fight the spread of viruses, influenza in particular, for at least a century. The modelling was presented as 'state of the art' science and ensured the modellers, too, significant broadcast airtime. But a critique of the models noted that they appear to be based on a 100-year-old model which may not understand the workings of the virus which causes Covid-19. (The SIR model[17] which is used was devised in the 1920s. Critics argue that it ignores scientific advances since then and that it therefore tends to overestimate the spread of the virus, which South African models are inclined to do.)[18] On one important issue – the wearing of masks – the initial scientific consensus was that they were needed only by health workers. This changed as scientists began to learn more about Covid-19 and they were later recognised as essential tools.[19] Perhaps most important of all, there was no cure or proven treatment for Covid-19 and so 'following the science' certainly did not mean simply making sure that infected people were given medicine which would ensure their recovery.

The limitations of 'the science' were also illustrated in early 2021, when vaccines which offered protection against Covid-19 became available. It quickly became common for scientists to win instant public acclaim by announcing research findings asserting the levels of protection offered by each vaccine. But the science was not quite as scientific as the national debate assumed. Vaccines are usually developed and tested over years, not months. Knowledge of the degree of protection they offer is generally gathered by experience and the vaccines adjusted accordingly. While most of the vaccines were subjected to thorough clinical trials, and all are safe, questions inevitably remained about how much protection they would offer in practice and how long they would last. While the difference between what the trials showed and what was likely to happen seemed marginal once vaccination began, the issue was complicated by the appearance of new strains of the virus and controversy over some of the vaccines' side effects.

In February 2021, trials assessing how effective the vaccine developed by Oxford University and manufactured by the pharmaceutical company AstraZeneca was against the new strain circulating in South Africa found that it gave little protection against mild and moderate disease. Plans to use the vaccine were dropped, causing controversy.[20] But, because the trials were only conducted among younger people, they did not test how effective the vaccines were at preventing severe disease or death among older people.[21] The trials were obviously useful in showing how the vaccine worked among a particular group of people. But, in addition to the South African decision to withdraw it, information gaps in the reports on clinical trials ensured that it was denied permission for use in Switzerland and approved only for people under age 65 in half a dozen European countries, not because it clearly would not help older people but because no one knew whether it would.[22] None of this showed that the science was flawed – it was as useful as it could be in the circumstances. But it did illustrate the point that there was very little undisputed 'science' on Covid-19 which the government could simply follow.

More important, there was no scientific consensus on how to deal with Covid-19. Another important difference between this virus and HIV is that the measures and behaviours necessary to avoid HIV did not require suspension of social, economic and religious life. Stemming Covid-19 did. This required policymakers and scientists to weigh up costs and benefits in a way not required by HIV and Aids. Inevitably, they reached different conclusions about how much freedom should be suspended to fight the virus. This was reflected not only in the view of a minority of scientists that few, if any, restrictions are needed,[23] but, among those who recognised the need for restrictions, on how extensive they should be and what goal they should serve (whether they should aim to stop transmission of the virus or merely to contain it).[24]

None of this meant, as the anti-common-sense lobby claimed, that science was simply a euphemism for prejudice. The protective measures were necessary, a reality which was to be demonstrated repeatedly during the fight against the virus. Nor did the fact that scientists changed their view on masks mean that they were charlatans who had no idea what they were doing: judgements which change as the evidence changes are the essence of science. That many scientists shifted their view on masks in response to evidence should, in principle, boost confidence since it showed that they were not ignoring evidence which contradicted their initial view. But these examples show that there was no settled, self-evident science which merely had to be followed to ensure safety and well-being.

It was noted in the Introduction that only medical science was regarded as science. The editorial in the *South African Medical Journal* mentioned earlier observed:

> In the absence of efficacious biomedical interventions against COVID-19, legal mechanisms and behavioural factors are central to bringing the COVID-19 pandemic under control. It is therefore unfathomable why experts who hail from the humanities and social sciences, or even relevant members of civil society and the private sector, have been deemed unworthy of MAC membership and irrelevant to the body's envisaged role of advising government.[25]

An effective response to the virus could not rely on technical medical solutions since there were none available until vaccines were developed. Stopping Covid-19's spread depended, therefore, on influencing human behaviour, and so knowledge of society and the perspectives of the key citizens' groups would be at least as valuable as the advice of medical scientists who, given Covid-19's novelty, had little science to offer. 'Following the science' really meant 'following what a selection of medical scientists believed the science to be'. And, in South Africa, it also seemed to mean taking seriously some knowledge but ignoring other varieties of knowledge which might be more valuable in protecting health and lives.

'Following the science' was not a straightforward – and self-evidently beneficial – choice because it begged the question of which science to follow. As some heated arguments between scientists confirm, there are competing 'sciences':[26] to follow one school is to ignore others. This is a choice and those who 'follow the science' are responsible for their choices. South Africa's government did not embrace the 'science' of those who dismissed the virus and the need to combat it. But it embraced a 'science' which was just as tendentious and which may also have worsened the spread of Covid-19.

SURRENDERING AT THE START

South African medical scientists disagreed loudly on some issues. But they (or at least all whose view was heard repeatedly by the lay public) agreed on one point which was presented to the society as an expression of 'the science' – despite the fact that it differed from the view of many scientists in other parts of the world.

In his first public statements on Covid-19, Karim, by then chair of the MAC, declared that it was 'inevitable that South Africa will experience a severe epidemic' because 'the rest of the world' had been unable to avoid it.[27] Preventive measures – the recently imposed lockdown – were needed not to prevent mass infections but to 'buy time' to make it more likely that the health system could cope with the cases it would inevitably be required to treat. So sure was he that many would fall severely ill and die that, in a much-quoted public briefing in April 2020, he listed as one stage in the country's response to Covid-19 'Bereavement and the Aftermath', which included 'expanding burial capacity'.[28]

The rationale for this view was not entirely clear. Karim's briefing, given a couple of weeks after the lockdown began, noted that the exponential increase in cases had been halted and that the curve plotting case numbers had almost flattened in the days after the lockdown was imposed. He declared that 'South Africa's epidemic trajectory is unique', despite the fact that one of his own slides showed that China and South Korea's curves had also flattened.[29] But he did not draw from this the apparent logical conclusion – that the promising beginning showed that the virus could be reduced to a minor threat. Despite the early success, the 'exponential spread' of the virus could not be prevented 'unless SA has a special protective factor ... not present anywhere else in the world'.[30]

This was not his view alone. All the medical scientists who weighed in on the public debate agreed that nothing could be done to prevent many people from falling ill and dying. Wits University's Madhi predicted in April 2020 that 25 000 people would die of Covid-19 during that year. He added that, while this seemed high, it was 'probably equal' to the number who died annually of tuberculosis (TB), 'which would never lead to a national lockdown'.[31] Ten months later, on 24 January 2021, Madhi marvelled at the low number of deaths and hospitalisations despite the fact that it was much higher than his original estimate: 'No-one could have predicted what happened in South Africa,' he said.[32] On the day he was thus quoted, 40 874 deaths from Covid-19 had been reported.[33] The SAMRC's excess deaths report, which measures how many more people died of natural causes than in previous years, reported 132 481 between 20 May 2020 and 30 January 2021.[34] So not only did he consider a death rate equal to the number who died of TB acceptable, he made the same claim about one which was one and a half to five times the number he estimated. Madhi did not say why he considered so high a death rate surprisingly low. Professor Marc Mendelson, the head of infectious diseases and HIV medicine at Groote Schuur Hospital, who has co-authored statements and articles with Madhi, insisted that 'sixty percent or so of our country will become infected over the next two years'.[35] There was a slight twist to Madhi and Mendelson's position, to which we will return, but they are united in assuming that large numbers of cases and deaths were inevitable.

The head of the SAMRC, Professor Glenda Gray, who achieved media celebrity by denouncing lockdown regulations, justified her opposition to restrictions in May 2020 thus:

With increasing knowledge of the virus, we now know that those most vulnerable are the elderly and those with comorbidities. However, people under 30, and school-going children are not. You don't put the whole country into lockdown because you don't know how to deal with [the] elderly and the people who have vulnerabilities. Non-pharmaceutical interventions should include targeted strategies to protect the vulnerable while those who would not be affected by the virus should be allowed back into society.[36]

The reporters who interviewed Gray seemed unaware – or chose not to point out – that her position in effect echoed the 'herd immunity' view which, from a very early stage of the pandemic, influenced government responses in the United Kingdom, Sweden and some states in the United States. It claims that, if a particular percentage of the population contracts a virus, it will be unable to spread further because it will run out of hosts. The virus should thus be allowed to spread to everyone except those who are vulnerable to severe illness and death.

In October 2020, three of its proponents issued the Great Barrington Declaration, named after a town in Massachusetts where they had gathered at a workshop hosted by the American Institute for Economic Research (AIER), a libertarian US think tank 'with the self-proclaimed agenda of promoting "personal freedom, free markets, private property, limited government, and sound money", and with a long record of attacking proponents of action on climate change'.[37] The three professors who authored it were taken to the Trump White House where their declaration was welcomed by the secretary for health and Trump's Covid-19 advisor.[38] Gray was later to claim that the government's restrictions were 'unscientific' but the scientists whose view she favoured seemed happy to see their stance sponsored and supported by the peddlers of right-wing 'anti-science'.

By early 2021, the countries in which versions of this approach exerted influence were among the worst affected in the world. The US's case and death numbers were the highest; in proportion to population, the United Kingdom was third worst (despite backing away from 'herd immunity' when it was told that this would incur crippling human costs[39]) and the United States was eighth out of 152 countries.[40] Sweden, whose population is around one-third of that of the Nordic region, reported infections, at the beginning of February 2021, which were two-thirds of those for the region; its cases were nearly double (180%) that of all its neighbours combined. Its death toll accounted for over three-quarters of Nordic fatalities, just under three and a half times the rest of the region combined.[41]

How scientific was this view? One of the declaration's authors' grasp of reality was so tenuous that they calculated 'a UK fatality rate so low that in fact it was mathematically impossible', while another claimed that 'real circulation of Covid was "waning fast" and that ... testing was just picking up "harmless virus particles"' – only a couple of months before Britain was engulfed in a second wave more damaging than the first.[42] This approach has been widely condemned by many scientists. They point out that 'herd immunity' theories claim that viruses will be unable to circulate if a particular percentage of the population is vaccinated, not that viruses should be left free to spread. Some also note that, even when vaccines are available, 'herd immunity' remains largely a theory since the only virus to ever be entirely eradicated is smallpox. Summing up some of their objections, Professor Kristian Andersen, an immunologist at the Scripps Research Institute in La Jolla, California, said that relying on 'herd immunity' would prompt a 'catastrophic' loss of human lives without necessarily speeding up society's return to normal: 'We have never successfully been able to do it before, and it will lead to unacceptable and unnecessary untold human death and suffering.'[43]

The Great Barrington Declaration's links to a right-wing think tank averse to measures which protect human health (and the planet) if they obstruct economic activity – and its embrace by the Trump administration – do not necessarily mean that those who endorse this view (which may well include Gray and other South African scientists) are themselves on the political right. But this 'science' is dubious – it ignores the fact that millions of people fall into vulnerable categories and so would need protecting, and does not say how that many people are to be kept out of harm's way while the virus is allowed to circulate freely. Gray did not say how some five million people in South Africa living with HIV and Aids were to be kept away from the rest of the population. This 'science' also took no account of the fact that many of the vulnerable are of working age – by 16 November, some 40 per cent of the people in South Africa who were reported to have died after testing positive were under the age of 60. Almost all were of working age, between 20 and 60,[44] so lives could be saved only by removing large numbers of people from economic activity. It also ignores the effect of 'long Covid' in which people who are no longer infected experience sometimes debilitating symptoms for months afterwards. One study in the US found that about 30 per cent of people who were infected experienced 'persistent' symptoms 'for as long as 9 months after illness'.[45] But, whatever the intentions of its authors, its key feature is that it elevates to a supreme goal the right of people to engage in economic activity and so is opposed by those who see the preservation of life and health as paramount. As will be seen, putting lives first also protects the economy. But that does not change the reality that Gray's view, so enthusiastically embraced by 'First World' South Africa, is not only a minority position among scientists elsewhere in the world but one which stems from a minority experience in South Africa, that of the suburbs, where restrictions are seen as an irksome constraint on economic and social life, not a key to preserving life and health.

While Gray seemed more willing to pin her public colours to this view, other scientists don't seem that far from it. Mendelson's reasons for saying that 60 per cent of the country would contract Covid-19 – a view which was echoed by Mkhize (see chapter 3) – were never reported. But there is a striking similarity between this calculation and that of the proponents of herd immunity: 'most models' expect some 60 to 70 per cent of the population to be infected before 'herd immunity' is achieved.[46] By insisting that the virus would continue to spread until that percentage was reached and that nothing could be done about it, Mendelson appears to have been advocating 'herd immunity' without saying so as explicitly as Gray. Madhi's view is also compatible with this approach. The view of the virus of South Africa's most revered scientists was also that which encouraged elites in countries whose approach invariably ensured more cases and deaths.

The government's response was different but similar. It maintained a lockdown in the face of objections from most of the scientists. But, following Karim's view, it did so not to stop Covid-19 but because it assumed that all that could be done was to slow the inevitable spate of illnesses to enable the health system to cope. This view was closer to that of the other scientists than their later squabbles would suggest – in his 2021 celebration of a death toll he, but surely no one who is not a medical scientist, considered small, Madhi mentioned low hospital admissions as a welcome, unexpected reality. Whatever their purported differences, they shared a common approach: that the virus could not be stopped or reduced to levels at which it was not a threat to many people.

'FIRST WORLD' VISION

The science journalist Laura Spinney argues that there is a 'cold war' between scientists across the globe who are divided into two camps on how to respond to the virus – those who want to eliminate it and those who want to suppress it.

She quotes the epidemiologist Michael Baker, who argued in early February 2021 that it was not too late to eliminate the virus rather than simply to keep it at bay. This would require burdensome restrictions but would yield much more benefit – short-term pain would ensure great longer-term benefits. He says that, in New Zealand, billionaires were persuaded to lobby the government to lock down early and hard to beat the virus. When he asked them why they did it, they replied: 'We didn't get filthy rich by not being good at assessing and managing risk.' Interestingly, among those who favour elimination, according to Spinney, is Nkengasong, head of the Africa CDC.[47] Others phrase this as a dispute between those who want merely to 'flatten' the curve of infections, keeping numbers steady enough to ensure that the health system can cope, and those who argue that several countries have shown that the curve could be 'smashed' or 'crunched', reducing cases to as close to zero as possible.[48]

The debate between South Africa's visible scientists was a little different: none were interested in eliminating the virus or 'smashing' the curve; the argument was between those who wanted to use restrictions to 'flatten' it so that the health system could cope and those who implied that even this was futile – as will be seen in chapter 3, the priority of all the scientists mentioned here bar Karim was to denounce the lockdown. Both camps' view was presented as 'the science' despite the fact that both their views were rejected by many scientists elsewhere. It was also accepted by the debate as 'the science' and quickly came to dominate the way in which media, citizens' organisations and the other voices which shape the public debate saw the pandemic. 'The restrictions are only meant to ready the health system' became a received wisdom. Other 'sciences' were available – they were simply ignored.

Nor did the position embraced by the scientists describe reality. It was simply not true that no country had avoided a severe epidemic. At the time Karim's presentation claimed this, the WHO reported that only 10 759 people had tested positive for Covid-19 in Africa[49] – since

2 415 of those cases were in South Africa, this meant that its 46 other member states had reported a little over 8 000 cases; to state the obvious, this was not a 'severe' epidemic. It was noted earlier that his own slides contained evidence of countries which were averting a severe epidemic. So 'the science' relied on the highly unscientific practice of ignoring evidence which did not support a theory.

What the 'First World' sees

Why would the scientific establishment be united behind a view which was contradicted by the daily news bulletins? After all, they presumably read the daily numbers from other countries which they were ignoring.

One possibility is that they knew that other countries had avoided severe epidemics but didn't believe that South Africa could do this. On what would they have based this judgement? The reasons would seem obvious: reports of the inadequacies of the public health system abound and many people live in poverty, which makes it more difficult for them to maintain distances from each other or to take other protective measures. But this 'common sense' view may also show two biases which weakened the country's response to Covid-19 – it assumes that a country's ability to control the virus depends on the strength of its health system, and that people living in poverty are unable (or unwilling) to protect themselves.

Assuming that countries with better health systems would be better able to deal with Covid-19 seems so obviously right that it could be seen as 'common sense'. But the 'common sense' view was already being contradicted when the scientists made claims which seemed to rely on it. By April, it had become clear that Italy, a country with more physicians per 1 000 people than South Korea, was battling to contain the virus while South Korea was largely keeping it at bay.[50] This told a bigger story – most of the countries which experienced the worst epidemics (the United States, the United Kingdom, Italy and France) were world leaders in medical expertise and technology. Why were they more affected than countries less endowed with both? Part of the answer may have been political – in the US (and Brazil) political leadership refused to take Covid-19 seriously; the UK arguably had the same problem although not in as extreme a form. But this did not explain all the cases.

A more general explanation is that these countries are expert in curative medicine, in how to treat already ill people and offer them the best hope of recovery. But there was no cure for Covid-19; it was not even clear how it should be treated. The initial response to the virus, consistent with the thinking on which curative medicine rests, was that ventilators were needed to assist severely ill patients who were unable to breath. It became routine in the early stages of the pandemic to note that particular countries (all of them, of course, in the 'Third World') owned a very small number of ventilators, which they would need to treat many people.[51] But this overestimated the ability of ventilators to save lives. In South Africa, according to Professor Ross Hofmeyr of Groote Schuur Hospital, 'As we moved into the surge of the pandemic, the survival rate for patients who needed mechanical ventilation was about 1 for every five or six patients.'[52] The hospital then used high-flow nasal oxygen, a less intrusive procedure, to treat patients and this increased the recovery rate, although ventilators are still used. Hofmeyr insisted that ventilators do save some lives, but their effect is limited.

Hofmeyr's comment is a rarity, a discussion by a South African medical scientist of the impact of hospital treatment on patients with Covid-19. The publication in which it appeared – published by two non-governmental organisations, Section 27 and the Treatment Action Campaign – was largely ignored by the mainstream media, which has not reported on the success rate of hospitals. Nor does the report say how many lives were saved – it says only that 'many successes' were achieved by this therapy. In South Africa and elsewhere, it is not clear how effective curative medicine is at assisting severely ill people infected by the virus. So, there is no hard evidence to support the 'common sense' assumption that the best way to fight Covid-19 was by ensuring that as many people as possible received the best curative medicine.

What does seem clear from the global evidence is that curative medicine is not as effective in combatting Covid-19 as public health measures which place prevention, not cure, at the centre. The study of South Korea and Italy argues that the former's superior ability to contain cases and deaths 'is partially due to the reactionary nature of Italy's public health measures compared to South Korea's proactive response'. While South Korea used 'technology and the holistic education of its physician community' to prevent infections,[53] Italy tried to fight the battle in the hospitals, which meant treating those who were already ill. Public health or preventive measures seem to have been far more effective at curbing Covid-19; countries which had limited curative health assets but experience in public health were better able to protect their population than those who relied on curative medicine. They included East Asian countries which had battled coronavirus epidemics and African countries which had to contend with epidemics such as Ebola.[54] The historian Florence Bernault, noting that Covid-19 has revived familiar images of Africa as a continent incapable of combatting disease, argues that Ebola is one of several epidemics which have been contained by preventive strategies in Africa:

> ... the history of epidemics and biomedicine demonstrates the long experience and extensive expertise of researchers, caregivers, and ordinary people. In addition, the experience of crises, especially health crises, is much stronger in Africa than in Western countries. What history and anthropology demonstrate is the importance of dialogue and mutual consultation between communities, experts

and researchers in the social sciences, and the need to trust local understanding and strategies.[55]

If South Africa's scientists believed that the inequities and weaknesses in its public health system made high case numbers inevitable, they were making a choice for curative rather than preventive medicine. They were also, Bernault suggests, choosing an inferior response partly because they were closed to the possibility that the rest of Africa may offer vital expertise. This is not surprising. 'First World' health-care facilities are a symbol of sophistication and progress. According to the anthropologist Alice Street, 'the development reputation of countries and regions in the poorer parts of the world [is] often read off the wall of their hospitals'.[56] In rural Indonesia, where she did her fieldwork, local bureaucrats, international donors and investors often used the quality of equipment and biomedical care at local hospitals as a primary indicator of development or modernity.[57] To excel at 'modern medicine' is to demonstrate civilisation, and this seems to have been important to South Africa's medical scientists – as it is to 'First World' South Africa.

But symbols of progress are not necessarily good at curing people infected with a new virus. To say that the priority is to ready the health system is to tell people to pin their hopes on hospital rather than on being protected from the virus. This is not purely a 'scientific' view: curative, technology-based medicine is seen as the only way to tackle illness in South Africa's 'First World' milieu because it is a sign of sophistication, not necessarily because it is what is needed. That the scientists share this bias seems likely, since they have spent their entire careers working within this view. Their attempt to press for treatment for everyone living with HIV and Aids was important and necessary. But the vigour with which they did this had much to do with the fact that curative medicine had found a way to reduce it to a chronic condition. Similarly, they loudly championed Covid-19 vaccines because these are born of the curative medicine in which they are steeped.

The claim that 'no country' had avoided a severe epidemic also showed a 'First World' bias. It was certainly true that no Western European or North American country avoided this (although some did much better than others). Since South Africa's medical scientists tend to pepper their discussions with references to the USA and Western Europe, it seems fair to assume that their thinking on the virus was drawn from their reading of those countries' experience.

There are interesting parallels between the South African scientific consensus and the view of the scientists who advised the British government:

> In early February 2020, UK advisers on the Scientific Advisory Group for Emergencies (Sage), against World Health Organization advice, took the view that coronavirus, like influenza, could not be stopped. Ignoring UK coronavirus experts and effective country responses in Asia, they followed the rulebook for pandemic influenza.[58]

They maintained this view despite the fact that, by March, it had become clear that five East Asian countries and New Zealand 'had largely contained the virus'. So had the Indian state of Kerala whose planning and quick action was widely hailed as an example to others.[59] Western academics and journalists, who find the idea of an Indian state governed by a left-wing alliance outperforming most of the 'First World' deeply disturbing, like to point out that its case numbers later increased significantly (because it hosts many migrants) and was at one point among the highest in India; it experienced high case numbers during India's 'second wave'. But, by February 2021, it had recorded only 4 105 deaths[60] out of a population of some 35 million.[61]

These countries and territories showed that Covid-19 could be effectively contained.

A year later, despite lockdowns and one of the highest death rates per million people in the world, these British scientists had not changed their position. The 'official scientists still insisted that the virus could not be suppressed' and that a combination of lockdowns and vaccination would merely reduce the damage it caused.[62] While South Africa has, throughout the pandemic, stressed its cooperation with the WHO, and its use of WHO scientists, the world body's position on this issue differed from that which guided the South African approach. The WHO director-general, Tedros Adhanom Ghebreyesus, warned in mid-March: 'The idea that countries should shift from containment to mitigation is wrong and dangerous.'[63] In other words, they should be 'smashing the curve' not 'flattening' it. In South Africa, 'science' is not what the WHO says it is but what a particular set of UK scientists said it was. This does not necessarily mean that South Africans were directly influenced by their UK counterparts. But it does suggest that they see the 'science' in much the same way.

The 'First World' bias is also revealed by scientists' attitudes towards the rest of the continent. Madhi's view that Africa may have been protected by 'poor conditions' was noted earlier. It is consistent with that of the BBC, which was eager to deny the possibility that African countries might have preventive health capacity. In an interview Karim gave to *Nature*, he acknowledged that hospitalisations and deaths were low in 'Africa' but added: 'I don't have the answer … At the moment, it's an enigma. The reason will reveal itself in due course.'[64] In an interview with the BBC he confessed to being 'all at sea' as he tried to make sense of this.[65]

Karim's candour is refreshing (and highly unusual among South African scientists – he is probably the only one who acknowledges error) but revealing. Like many of his colleagues, he refers to Africa as a distant, exotic terrain. The stock response of an epidemiologist puzzled by the progression of an epidemic in other countries would surely be to consult colleagues there. This seems not to have occurred to him despite the fact that he chairs the Joint United Nations Programme on HIV/AIDS (UNAIDS) Scientific Expert Panel and belongs to WHO committees. (Revealingly, he also belongs to the US National Academy of Medicine, the American Academy of Microbiology and the Association of American Physicians.[66]) This international scientific figure apparently either knows of no colleague elsewhere on the continent or, more likely, does not believe those he does know worth consulting. There is nothing in these responses to distinguish the speaker from an American or European scientist musing on the latest mystery to emerge from 'the dark continent'.

Vision of poverty, poverty of vision

There is a second possible reason for the judgement that a severe epidemic was inevitable despite the fact that it was avoided elsewhere – the view that 'Third World' South Africa was incapable of protecting itself from a severe outbreak.

This was a common, probably overwhelming view in 'First World' South Africa, reflected repeatedly in public discussion. Just as it was assumed that Africa was incapable of protecting itself from the virus, so Africans who lived in South Africa's townships and shack settlements, its 'Third World', were assumed to be similarly incapable. An oft-cited reason was overcrowding, poverty and even the absence of clean water. It was also true, although less frequently commented upon, that most people in these areas relied for their transport on minibus taxis (used by an estimated 69 per cent of commuters[67]) in which the virus was likely to spread, particularly if drivers did not open all windows or limit passenger numbers. One reason why women suffered disproportionately from Covid-19 is that they use taxis more frequently than men.[68] But 'First World' South Africa did not see these realities as challenges to be overcome in partnership with the people who lived in these areas. If the government's approach to restrictions is a guide, it was assumed that people in 'Third World' South Africa were both incapable of protecting themselves, and unwilling to do this.

It soon became clear that the government had a low opinion of the 'Third World' citizens whose votes keep it in office. After the lockdown began, the minister responsible for implementing the regulations, Nkosazana Dlamini Zuma, partly justified a ban on the sale of tobacco products by warning that 'our people', code for poor, black people, tended to share cigarettes.[69] Minister Ebrahim Patel justified a ban on the sale of cooked food by warning that people in low-income areas bought cooked meat from roadside stalls;[70] a ban on alcohol sales was said to prevent people engaging in drunken violence and so overburdening the health system.[71] A rule banning outdoor exercise after 9am was justified as an attempt to prevent people wandering in public.[72] As will be seen, these and other regulations enraged suburban opinion and were cited frequently as evidence of the irrationality of the restrictions introduced to slow the virus's spread. But, as the ministerial statements show, their purpose was not to prevent suburbanites smoking on porches, sipping cocktails, ordering sushi or walking dogs. It was to prevent assumed outbreaks of irresponsibility among the township poor.

Nor did the government trust the townships to abide by the rules. Some 73 000 troops were deployed on the streets to help police enforce them,[73] further confirmation that the authorities believed that townships needed to be forced to be safe. Almost inevitably, imposing the rules in this way ensured that their residents would face a threat to their safety other than the virus. Anger at the military's role in policing the rules was triggered by the killing of Collins Khosa, a resident of Alexandra township, by soldiers on Good Friday, 10 April, after they found him drinking beer in his yard.[74] The rules said people could not buy alcohol or drink it in bars or taverns, not that they could not drink it in their homes. This was not the only incident in which soldiers were accused of bullying residents, although it became a symbol for the others. The fact that the government committee responsible for the Covid-19 rules was the Command Council, showed that the government had convinced itself that it was waging a war – against, it seemed, its own electorate.

How accurate was this assumption of 'Third World' ignorance and indifference in contrast to 'First World' awareness and sophistication? Alcohol does fuel violence, largely in low-income areas, which does place pressure on hospitals. While the suburbs are hardly vice-free, affluence enables residents to keep the consequences of their indulgences (mainly) out of the casualty wards. But the assumption that people living in poverty are ignorant or irresponsible is dubious – they may have been more concerned to protect themselves than the suburbs. Media coverage of township areas revealed that many people wore masks and often complained that they were being forced to queue for groceries (or food parcels) in circumstances which made distancing difficult. Unintendedly revealing evidence that township residents were more inclined to welcome restrictions than suburbanites was offered by two American scholars' study on township attitudes to the virus, which found that people were so worried about their physical health that they told interviewers that restrictions would not impair their mental health. In a remarkable example of the condescension of the global 'First World', the authors used this evidence of support for measures which fought the virus to scold township residents for their ignorance of mental health.[75] 'Third World' citizens, it seems, place an excessive value on life and health rather than mental well-being. There is also copious evidence of deep-seated fears of riding in taxis.[76] When schools reopened, many of the people who were assumed not to know or care about Covid-19 were reluctant to send their children back to the classroom for fear of spreading the virus.[77] Suburban residents, by contrast, flocked back to restaurants when infection levels remained reasonably high.

Given these attitudes, there does seem a more than reasonable prospect that, had the government engaged with the townships and shack settlements on ways to protect people which recognised the realities of life in these areas, a productive partnership might have emerged. In theory, the government response seemed to be aware of, and interested in, working with people at the grassroots. In his April 2020 presentation, Karim declared that 'South Africa has a unique component to its response, i.e. active case finding'. He added: 'Only South Africa has more than 28 000 community health workers going house-to-house in vulnerable communities for screening and testing to find cases.'[78] Besides placing testing and tracing at the heart of the response, a point to which this book will return, this seemed to recognise the need to engage people in protecting themselves. But government employees knocking on doors to screen and test is not an acknowledgement of citizens as active partners, even if they are called 'community' health workers. It is simply another way in which the government tells people what to do.

The scientists showed no interest in partnership with most South Africans. They said little about the need to provide washing stations for people lacking water – an idea implemented in some African countries[79] – even though this response was piloted in South Africa.[80] Nor did they offer suggestions for protecting people who live in overcrowded homes. Some did tell journalists that overcrowding in taxis was a health hazard, but only so that they could denounce the lockdown.[81] And so, it seems likely that their assumption that the country would not be able to contain the spread of the virus was based less on a recognition of the conditions of people living in poverty than the belief that only technological medical solutions could deal with the problem and that people living in poverty did not know how to protect themselves or did not care.

The scientists saw 'the science' as they did because, as products of the internal 'First World', it was the only 'science' they could see.

TESTING AND TRACING: DIFFERENT BUT THE SAME

The next chapter explores the ways in which the attitudes discussed here made high numbers of cases and deaths inevitable. But one aspect must be discussed here because it shows how wedded the scientists were to the curative medicine of the 'First World'.

It was noted earlier that Madhi and Mendelson, while endorsing the South African scientific consensus that a severe epidemic was inevitable, seem to have been the only two to identify problems in testing and tracing and to insist that these needed to be addressed. In a Guest Editorial in the *South African Medical Journal* in June[82] (and an abbreviated version in *The Conversation* in May[83]), they identified the failure of the test and trace programme and urged a new approach. This suggested that at least some South African medical scientists were able to remove their gaze from Europe and the United States long enough to see other realities.

But their view repeats the consensus. We would expect scientists who saw that the testing and tracing programme was not working to suggest ways in which it could be made to work since it was the key weapon of countries which had effectively 'contained' Covid-19, to use the WHO's language. They argue, rather, that testing and tracing cannot stem the virus. It should rather be used for hospitalised patients, to allow 'optimal clinical and infection prevention management of suspected severe COVID-19, and patient flow to enable hospitals to cope with escalating numbers'[84] – in other words, to enable hospitals to manage their treatment better. It should also be used for health-care workers with symptoms and their contacts 'to limit hospital outbreaks and protect the integrity of the health service', and staff and patients in 'long-term care facilities, which international studies indicate are hotspots for outbreaks'. 'Other essential services personnel' could also be tested and their contacts traced.[85]

The authors do not recommend testing and tracing to contain the virus in the general population because they do not believe that it can do this. In their discussion of why testing and tracing did not work, they note that South Africa 'is dependent on foreign companies for testing materials and kits, for which there is a high demand globally, leading to serious shortages'.[86] Even if the 'turnaround time' problem were solved, so that test results emerged far quicker from the laboratory, field workers who administer tests could not reach enough people to keep track of patients. In any event, 50 to 80 per cent of people who are infected show no symptoms and so would not be identified for testing. Identifying only a quarter of cases, tracing contacts and isolating them 'could assist in slowing the rate of (not preventing) community transmission of the virus and mitigate to some extent the anticipated surge in severe Covid-19 cases occurring over a very short period of time. By doing so, healthcare facilities may be somewhat better equipped to deal with the anticipated surge of Covid-19 cases.'[87] But, while this might have been achievable in the early phases of the pandemic, it was now unrealistic because there were too many cases to trace. So, 'the strategy of actively searching for infectious cases is now likely to yield little value, and … there is acceptance that transmission will be ongoing (and will not be reversed by going back into a harsher lockdown).'[88] Since testing and tracing would not protect against the virus, the consensus route forward – handwashing, mask-wearing and distancing to keep numbers down to protect the health service – was the most workable strategy.

This is not an alternative to the mainstream view. It does not see testing and tracing as a way to 'smash the curve'. At best, it may be yet another weapon in the quest to ready the always-central health system, not a means to join those countries which contained the virus. And even that is not possible because the case numbers are too high and most people who contract the virus don't show symptoms. The proposed remedy is useful only for a very select group of people.

Predictably, with the exception of the throwaway line about essential workers, the criterion for selecting beneficiaries is the familiar goal, making the health system work. (Even health workers seem to be selected not because people on the front line of the fight against disease need protecting but 'to protect the integrity of the health system'.)

Madhi's support for this position is particularly odd since he was a co-author of an article in April by a group of University of the Witwatersrand academics urging the government to adopt the South Korean approach by giving priority to testing and tracing.[89] This was the only contribution to the public debate of the sort – a call to use test and trace to reduce cases and deaths. Predictably, given the attitude of the debate, it was ignored. But, given Madhi's position in the later article, it appears that the only medical scientist to publicly support this view recanted not much later. (Madhi may have co-authored because the article also urged an end to the lockdown – but its proposed alternative is very different to the one he endorsed shortly afterwards.)

There are some obvious objections to this view. One is that the authors' claim that 50 to 80 per cent of infected people have no symptoms is contested by other scientists. Dr Anthony Fauci, director of the USA's National Institute of Allergy and Infectious Diseases, believes that the figure is 40 to 45 per cent.[90] South Korean estimates put the proportion at 20 to 30 per cent in the 'first wave' of the virus, 40 per cent by the end of November.[91] Even the source on which they rely is much more tentative than they claim: it says that this 'may' be the proportion, not that it is.[92] (Fittingly perhaps, the lead author of the article they cite, Carl Heneghan, is also an author of the Great Barrington Declaration.) So, patients without symptoms appear to be far less an obstacle to testing than they suggest. And why did this constraint not prevent testing and tracing working effectively in East Asia, Australia and New Zealand (and in parts of Africa too)?

More generally, the argument confuses cause and effect. It says that test and trace cannot work because case numbers are too high;

many of their colleagues elsewhere in the world would insist that the numbers are high because test and trace did not work. These scientists agree that the purpose of restrictive measures (which include, but are not restricted to, lockdowns) is not to make the virus disappear because that is beyond their power. But nor is its aim to 'ready the health system'. It is to reduce numbers so that it is possible to test infected people and trace their contacts with a view to stopping the spread of the virus, which is precisely what countries which kept cases and deaths low did.[93] If test and trace was not working, the logical response was to tighten restrictions to get case numbers low enough to allow it to work. The authors simply dismiss this, predictably since they are vociferous opponents of lockdown restrictions. In May, Mendelson insisted that the lockdown should be reduced to its lowest level immediately because it was 'doing more harm than good' but did not say what harm it was doing.[94] He claimed that 'the only countries which successfully flattened the curve through lockdown were those who were able to swiftly test, trace and quarantine on a mass scale.'[95] This ignores the fact that some countries kept numbers low enough to allow test and trace to work to 'smash', not 'flatten', the curve. But this admission by a South African scientist that testing, tracing and quarantining measures could succeed was followed not by a call that the country improve all three, but that it sharply limit their use.

His response is rare among South African medical scientists since it acknowledges a role for testing and tracing while the others either don't suggest any remedy – it is common to exhort people to 'live with the virus', ignoring the fact that many are dying from it – or fall back on remedying the health system. But even this sally into the debate is far more interested in the health system than in defeating the virus, to the extent of reducing health workers to objects which must be protected only because this will help 'the health system'. Whatever their differences in detail, the scientists were unanimous: nothing could be done to prevent many illnesses and deaths. At best, public health measures could protect the health system and, in theory, a small group of people who are considered particularly at risk. 'Following the science' did not mean, as it did when HIV and Aids stalked the land, giving priority to the saving of human life. It meant, rather, a fatalism which turned out to be self-fulfilling because, if policy does not give priority to preserving health and life, it is unrealistic to expect it to do that.

LOOKING WEST – AND LOOKING DOWN

So, the scientists' view is not 'the science'. It is the 'science' of a few.

There was no reason in theory why some local scientists could not have agreed with colleagues elsewhere who favoured swift and vigorous public health measures designed to suppress the virus. But the 'war' between contending views which Spinney noticed never reached South Africa.[96] Explicitly or implicitly, scientists here opted for the views of colleagues in the West who dismissed public health measures which hampered the economy or the lifestyles of the affluent and the middle class. While much lip service was paid to the importance of the WHO, at least by the government and Karim, there seemed no enthusiasm for the 'contain, don't mitigate' approaches of the global body and some of the strategies which went with it, such as a strong stress on testing and tracing and helping people living in poverty to protect themselves.

While everything the scientists said was treated with awe by the debate, they were, through 2020, fractious and given at times to arguing – as will be seen, arguments over the lockdown were debates between scientists as well as between them and the government.[97] So serious was the conflict between some scientists, all of whom served on the MAC, that the Bhekisisa Centre for Health Journalism published an article on the conflicts. Its author, Mia Malan, wrote:

> ... place a bunch of A-rated scientists on the same committee, many who are conducting COVID-19 research of their own and are therefore competing for funding and recognition, and you're heading for trouble. Add a disease for which there is no cure or treatment, a lack of clear scientific guidance and a government reluctant to release data that committee members are demanding, and the problem gets more complex.[98]

In Malan's view, based not only on the debates over Covid-19, but her time covering HIV and Aids, disputes between medical scientists, spurred not only by differences of opinion but also by professional rivalries, were as much a part of scientific life as laboratory experiments and peer reviewed articles. That every one of these scientists, while disagreeing on other issues, endorsed a version of 'the science' which was highly contested elsewhere, including in the United States and the United Kingdom, the countries which dominated discussion of the virus, is remarkable. Despite the 'war' Spinney describes, only one view prevailed in South Africa.

The reason surely lay in a simple reality – all the scientists are firmly embedded in 'First World' South Africa. If only curative medicine works, a severe epidemic was inevitable if there was no cure, particularly since countries which, in this view, are the centres of medical excellence, were struggling. This was doubly likely since most of the population were trapped in the 'Third World'. The government and the politicians, media, academics and citizens' organisations which shape the public debate accepted this version for the same reasons. As chapter 1 showed, they are, despite their many differences, embedded in 'First World' South Africa which talks about most South Africans incessantly but listens to them never, in which curative medicine, a suburban lifestyle and all the assumptions that accompany it are assumed to be signs of civilisation and what the fight against apartheid was meant to enable all to achieve. Given this, it is no surprise that alternative views within the country were not refuted but ignored, much as the babbling of a child trying to enter an adult conversation might be (not once during 2020 did either the medical scientists or the mainstream debate respond to the argument made here, even though it was widely published).

South Africa's elites chose one 'science' over others which might have offered an alternative to mounting case numbers and fatalities. They did this not because the medical scientists were persuaded, after careful thought, of the merits of a particular argument and the rest of the elite bowed to their expertise. The far more credible explanation is that they adopted, without much reflection at all, the view which we would expect from professionals in a country divided into two realities, and in which the national debate reflects the experiences and attitudes of the 'First World' minority, not the 'Third World' majority.

CHAPTER
3

The Science Unravels

The sense that the government and scientists are working together to fight a threat is meant to instil in citizens confidence and hope and to encourage them to support the battle against the common danger. In South Africa, this unity lasted all of a few weeks.

Initially, the public debate rallied around the common effort. We don't know how most citizens felt because in a country divided into two worlds, most of the country is not heard. But, among those whose voices are heard, there were few, if any, dissenting voices when the government declared the state of disaster and then imposed a lockdown on 27 March 2020, three weeks after the first case was reported. Organised business pledged support for the campaign against the virus despite the fact that economic activity would be curtailed. This goodwill was enhanced by relief that the government was listening to 'the science' and was not pursuing a 'political agenda'.

This support for official efforts to fight the virus was fairly common across the planet. What made it unusual in South Africa was that, for the past decade, the government and the debate has been at war and so the voices that are heard rarely if ever supported anything it did. The complicated nature of South Africa's divisions means that conflict within the 'First World' between the government and the insiders is suspended during national sporting events such as the 2010 football World Cup or the national rugby team's World Cup victories, the most recent of which had occurred only a few months before the lockdown. For a while, the debate seemed to have decided that the virus, too, required some temporary harmony prior to the resumption of hostilities.

This atmosphere prevailed despite the fact that restrictions were severe. The government's 'risk adjusted strategy' introduced five levels of lockdown, of which level 5 was the strictest – it began at this level. Like many other countries, it imposed bans on movement within the country as well as between it and other countries and closed all businesses except those which offered 'essential services'. No movement outside homes was allowed unless the movers were essential workers or could show they were on their way to buy necessities or seek medical help. It banned the sale of tobacco products and alcohol, and food stores were forbidden to sell cooked food.[1] Initially, this won wide acceptance although the government's troop deployments showed that it was not relying on goodwill alone in 'Third World' living areas.

The honeymoon lasted around three weeks. The first lockdown was imposed until 16 April and it seems to have been assumed by many in business and the suburbs that 'normal' life would resume on 17 April. When the restrictions were extended, the brief moment of national unity ended. Confirmation that the suburbs were no longer willing to endure restrictions to fight the virus came on 26 April. A survey commissioned by two newspapers, *City Press* and *Rapport*, found that 'strong' support for the lockdown had dropped from 77 per cent when it was first introduced, to 70 per cent when it was extended from 16 April to 30 April. While this was not a huge shift, it claimed too that only 38 per cent of people who responded wanted the lockdown extended beyond 30 April. It noted that these negative attitudes coincided with an announcement by Ramaphosa that the lockdown level would be reduced to 4, so easing some of the restrictions, and that he had also announced a R500 billion relief package to enable citizens to cope with the economic hardship wrought by the lockdown.[2]

Two points about the survey and the manner in which it was reported are important. On the latter, both *City Press*, the newspaper which reported it, and a representative of Victory Research, the company which conducted it, exaggerated the degree of public disaffection which the research claimed to reveal. The newspaper's headline claimed that South Africans were 'gatvol' (fed up) with lockdown; Ryan Coetzee of Victory Research said that 'the majority of citizens were now faced with the socioeconomic challenges of living in confinement, which made it difficult to continue supporting the measure.'[3] But this was not necessarily what the findings said. The drop from 77 to 38 per cent was among those who 'strongly supported' the lockdown, leaving open the possibility that a great many more supported it, albeit not strongly. Oddly, they did not say how many were in this category. They did say that 43 per cent were 'strongly opposed' to the lockdown continuing, which left open the possibility that a majority supported the measure. The survey also found that 71 per cent 'strongly supported' the alcohol ban and 65 per cent the ban on tobacco sales. It reported approval rates of 67 per cent for the president and 63 per cent for the minister of health; it said that 56 per cent had faith in the government's ability to control the pandemic but added that this view had majority support among black respondents but not among whites.[4]

This suggests a far more complicated (and less coherent) picture than the one presented by the commissioning newspaper or the research company. It is also strange that the findings were reported in a way which implies that people either 'strongly' support or oppose an action and that there are no views in between. The fact that these ambiguous findings were presented as a ringing rejection of the lockdown raises at least the possibility that this was less a test of public opinion than an attempt to influence it. Coetzee is a former senior Democratic Alliance (DA) strategist and the company's chief executive officer was Gareth van Onselen, who had also worked for the DA and whose previous post was at the South African Institute of Race Relations (SAIRR). The director of SAIRR, Dr Frans Cronje, had, as early as 2 April, within the first week of the lockdown, wanted the government to 'get as much economic activity back on track as soon as possible'[5] and later considered joining a legal action against the lockdown rules and their manner of enforcement.[6] Polling is not a neutral activity: some polls are conducted in the hope of influencing opinion; pollsters and those who commission them may also interpret their findings in ways which reflect their view of the world.

The accuracy of the poll is also open to question on two grounds. First, there is no way of checking how accurate broad surveys of public opinion are: how could we ever check how many people support a lockdown? But there is one type of polling which can be tested – that which measures party support before elections. Where polls which make claims about public opinion are conducted by pollsters who also poll party support, a rough and ready test of accuracy is how well they did at testing that support. While the method is hardly foolproof, it is reasonable to assume that pollsters who can accurately gauge the parties people support are far more likely to measure how they feel about lockdowns, or any other issue.[7] Van Onselen did poll the 2019 election on behalf of the SAIRR; his numbers were enough off the mark to prompt him to issue a lengthy statement trying to explain this.[8] Secondly, the poll was conducted during the lockdown and so respondents were not questioned face to face. According to Victory Research, it was conducted using a 'random digital dialling design' which presumably means that it was a telephone poll. This makes its claim that it was 'representative of the country's demographics'[9] open to challenge since phone polls tend to skew the sample in favour of more affluent voters (coverage of cellular phones in South Africa is very high but poor people tend to own phones which are far less likely to turn up in the data). While the poll may have reflected the country's racial and gender composition, it is hard to see how a telephone poll conducted in the midst of a pandemic could claim to have adequately polled the views of 'Third World' South Africa.

The survey's publication does seem to have been something of a turning point. It was widely quoted in the media and, from then on, it became increasingly common, in both traditional and digital media, to see lockdown measures as a constraint on the economy and on citizens' freedom rather than a necessary measure. It is of some importance to know whether this reflected a change in majority sentiment or only among opinion-makers and in the suburbs. Or, to put the point another way, whether it reflected what everyone thought or what 'First World' citizens thought. The evidence suggests that it reflected the concerns of the 'First World', as the South African debate always does.

What is clear is that, from then onwards, the residents of the suburbs – the 'First World' – became increasingly alienated from the lockdown and, more generally, from the government's attempt to follow its understanding of 'the science'. Middle-class resentment seems to have reached its breaking point in May when Ramaphosa, in an address further easing the restrictions, announced that cigarette sales could resume, only to backtrack after Dlamini Zuma (who has campaigned against smoking since she served as health minister in the 1990s) insisted that 'public opinion' (which she had manufactured by encouraging anti-smoking groups to complain) was opposed to tobacco and cigarette sales.[10] Anger was mixed with ridicule when the government allowed the sale of winter clothing but published regulations specifying in comic detail which items could be sold.[11] Ironically, there is evidence that retailers (who, like other businesses, are rarely laughed at by the debate) played a major role in writing the maligned rules, but this was never reported.[12]

Given the nature of South Africa's divisions, it does not seem fanciful to suggest that middle-class anger was at least partly a product of a sense among some white South Africans that a largely black government had no business telling them when they could drink, smoke, take walks or go to work. What is certain is that the 'First World' was not going to be told what to do by a government they (inaccurately) associated with the 'Third'.

THE SCIENCE OF THE SUBURBS

The scientists' truce with the government did not last much longer than that of the suburbs.

In May, with the fight against the virus only a couple of months old, some of them began an assault on the lockdown. The charge was led by Gray, who found herself embroiled in a public dispute with the minister of health. But she was not alone. Madhi and Mendelson joined in – we have seen that the latter wanted to move to virtually no restrictions at the height of the pandemic. They were joined by Dr Aslam Dasoo, convenor of the Progressive Health Forum. Karim did not join the anti-lockdown campaign – he was identified with the government position and the ensuing conflict seems to have largely inspired Malan's article cited in chapter 2. The dispute was complicated by the fact that all the participants were members of the MAC but seemed unable to agree on how it and the government had engaged with each other. But, while this clash prompted much media excitement, the two sides were not only members of the same committee. They agreed that trying to prevent a severe epidemic was futile.

Gray's attack, mentioned in chapter 2, was launched in mid-May. She labelled the government's decision to gradually withdraw from lockdown 'nonsensical and unscientific'. Many lockdown regulations were 'merely thumbsucks'. She added: 'We are seeing children for the first time with malnutrition [at Chris Hani Baragwanath Academic Hospital] … We have not seen malnutrition for decades and so we are seeing it for the first time in the hospital.' Like much of the national debate, she focused on the clothing regulations which were 'not based on science'. Also: 'In the face of a young population, we refuse to let people out. We make them exercise for three hours a day and then complain that there is congestion in this time. We punish children and kick them out of school and we deny them education. For what? Where is the scientific evidence for that?' Initially there had been good reason to implement the lockdown to buy time to ready the health system but this was 'largely achieved'. Another two weeks of lockdown 'may have supported the work that had been started and was critical' but its continuation ignored science and was 'nonsensical'. She argued for targeted strategies for the vulnerable while those 'not affected by the virus should be allowed into society'. 'With increasing knowledge of the virus, we know that those most vulnerable are the elderly and those with comorbidities. However, people under 30 and school going children are not.' She said the government had failed 'to understand the psyche of the populace.'[13] The article reporting her view also contained Mendelson's view that the lockdown should be dropped to level 1, the level at which the least restrictions applied.

Dasoo waded into the controversy much later. In an interview in October which stressed his role in the fight against medical apartheid and his African National Congress (ANC) membership, he complained about the 'fear and war talk' which was being used to describe the pandemic. He added, 'A national command council for a bloody virus? It's a lockdown committee. This is no war. This is a public health emergency.' It had 'given control to politicians, when health experts should have made the decisions'. The health system, he claimed, was 'decrepit' because 'politicians have for too long interfered in health-care decision-making'. Scientists had 'advised the government to implement a gradual lockdown' and had merely suggested stopping mass gatherings. They wanted the economy kept open because the poor had no means to store food. Instead, the government had closed schools, a measure against which he campaigned. The lockdown was not needed to prepare the health system: 'That was a soundbite. The health system was ramping up week by week.' Extending the lockdown beyond three weeks was a 'bad political decision' which 'reversed economic gains.'[14]

In response to Gray, Karim said the government had not ignored scientific advice. Another member of the MAC, Professor Ian Sanne, offered a more ambiguous reply. He said it was asked to 'advise on a risk adjusted approach to focus on hotspots, a screening and testing strategy and, in turn lockdown'. He added: 'We were asked about the approach, not the trigger levels and relationships to economic activity. We were informed that this would in future be used to determine the lockdown and economic activity in areas where Covid-19 is less. And that we agreed with.'[15] This means that the scientists were asked for a general approach, not to tell the government when to move from one lockdown level to another. What is not clear is what, according to Sanne, was agreed. His comment, as reported, could mean either that the scientists agreed that they should simply discuss a broad strategy or that they agreed on a specific strategy. But, although he too complained that the 'extended lockdown' was having a negative effect on the health system, his remarks do not seem to support Gray's claim (supported later by Dasoo) that the government ignored the scientists.

Mkhize offered a more detailed response to Gray in a media release. He insisted that the government did listen to the scientists. The MAC had presented the government with 50 advisory opinions, all of which it accepted. Its lockdown decisions were, he said, taken with the science in mind. The previous week, he added, Gray, who was chair of the MAC's Research Committee, was part of a team which was preparing an advisory on the lockdown – it had not yet been presented to him when she chose to speak to the media. As head of the SAMRC, she enjoyed access to the department but had never raised her concerns with it. He labelled her language as 'unprofessional and unbecoming' – a reference to her claims that the government was 'sucking' regulations 'out of its thumb' and that its rules were 'rubbish'. Divergent views from scientists were welcome but he urged them to avoid 'potentially destructive behaviour' and to engage 'constructively' with the government. The statement also took issue with Gray's claim about malnutrition – he noted that the number of cases at the hospital had reduced since the lockdown began 'when compared to the previous 4 years'. The statement also replied to a bizarre line of media questioning which demanded to know why he had appointed Karim and not Gray as chair of the MAC. He stated 'the obvious', which is that the minister was entitled to choose his own MAC chair, and added that nothing disqualified Karim from the post.[16]

Gray responded by complaining that she was being 'singled out'. She said she was not criticising the lockdown or its extension, only the regulations, and that she was speaking in her 'personal capacity', not as head of the SAMRC.[17] She did not take issue with Mkhize's claim that 50 advisories had been accepted and that she had not raised the issue with the ministry or department. She had already retracted her claim about malnutrition cases at Baragwanath. The SAMRC agreed to a health ministry request that it hold an inquiry into her conduct[18] but announced the next day that she had spoken in her personal capacity and that she had not breached its policies.[19] The inquiry was, therefore, abandoned before it began. Despite this distinct lack of persecution, she became an instant martyr.

Almost immediately after the acting director-general of health, Dr Anban Pillay, asked the MRC to investigate her, a group of medical and social scientists headed by Professor Adam Habib, vice-chancellor of the University of the Witwatersrand, rushed to her aid: they upheld 'the right to academic freedom of speech' and called on the government to 'engage openly with alternative views'.[20] A media article by Mark Heywood, a civil society activist, added that it was 'right' to defend Gray's freedom of speech but also important to 'be concerned that some of the underlying issues Gray and other health experts were raising are not getting the same attention. One of these is access to sufficient food and nutrition, hunger, and its impact on health and inequality.'[21] Gray declared herself 'grateful' to the SAMRC board and 'all those who have reached out to me personally during this unfortunate and trying time and especially to those who insisted on upholding the principles of academic freedom, which can only be of benefit to our country and all its people.'[22] She ended the year as Society Newsmaker of the Year, anointed by a business publication in a report so fawning that it would not have been out of place in the official media of a dictatorship. It said she had 'said what everyone was thinking.'[23]

The great lockdown controversy ended the largely artificial period of harmony between the government on the one hand, and the scientists (with the partial exception of Karim, who did not publicly defend the lockdown but did not attack it either), the suburban middle class and the media which largely acts as its voice on the other.[24] The claim that the government had ignored the advice of scientists became a theme, with others joining the chorus. In August, when Mkhize released 45 MAC advisories, noting that all but fewer than 5 per cent had been implemented 'in their entirety', the media latched onto the fact that the government had ignored a recommendation that minibus taxis operate at a maximum of 70 per cent capacity, allowing them to operate at 100 per cent instead.[25] This did not contradict Mkhize's earlier claim that all the advisories had been accepted since it came much later (he would presumably not have released them if it did) but the 'revelation' was seized on with gusto, much as a major expose might be. Clearly, a 'Third World' government had no business disagreeing with anything 'First World' scientists said, even if it had been elected by the majority of voters. It also illustrated that 'First World'

South Africa saw the pandemic through lenses which made high case numbers and fatalities inevitable.

The views of Gray, Dasoo and other lockdown opponents were treated by the media and the public debate as 'the science' despite (or because of) the fact that much of it seemed more like thinly disguised suburban prejudice. Its advocates were never slow to unfurl anti-apartheid credentials if they could, presumably to indicate that they were speaking 'for' not 'about' the majority of South Africans. But participation in the fight against apartheid does not inoculate against a suburban view of the world, whether it is held by scientists or cabinet ministers.

Gray's celebrated assault sounds more like the many attacks by suburbanites who assailed the government on digital media than a scientific analysis. Her proposed remedies showed that she remained firmly embedded in the Great Barrington Declaration's view of the pandemic, in which only 'the vulnerable' were protected and everyone else could behave as they pleased. Many scientists in other parts of the world would regard this view as 'unscientific and nonsensical'. Her insistence that schools open because pupils were immune from serious illness ignored evidence that people of school-going age have died of the disease.[26] In the view of one medical scientist, transmission in schools in Britain 'was likely crucial in the emergence of the more transmissible and dangerous variant' of the virus which ravaged that country.[27] Gray also seemed unaware that learners might take the virus home to family members, some of whom might be very vulnerable. The 'increasing knowledge of the virus' which she invoked is rejected by many scientists.

Nor was her account particularly coherent. She said 'the elderly' and those with comorbidities should be protected but those under 30 should not. Besides the fact that she did not say how they should be protected, what about the large section of the population over 30 but not elderly (and who may have no comorbidities which had yet been detected)? Were they to be protected and, if so, how? Were they to be left to protect themselves and, if so, why? She seemed unable to make up her mind about whether the lockdown should have lasted three weeks or five or to say why either was appropriate. The claim that she was drawing the country's attention to hunger and inequality bordered on the comic since her only comment on this issue was a factually incorrect claim about malnutrition which was ignorant of the realities facing people living in poverty. Nor did anyone who commented seem to notice that the head of the country's official medical research institute was unaware of realities in Soweto which would surely be known to most medical students.

The nature of Gray's complaint may well be revealed by her claim that the government had misread the 'psyche of the populace'. Since the only evidence of grassroots' attitudes we have suggests that people in townships did not share her unhappiness with the restrictions (hence the American researchers' disappointment at their failure to express distress), 'the populace' Gray had in mind was presumably her fellow suburbanites. She was indeed, as her praise poem in the business newspaper insisted, saying what 'everyone' thought – if 'everyone' is understood to mean everyone who would normally be encountered at a suburban social occasion.

Dasoo's 'science' did identify an important flaw in the government approach – the attempt to militarise control of the virus, which cost lives and triggered abuses. The term 'command council' sounded authoritarian and implied a degree of power which the government never had. But no medical training was needed to say what many public commentators with no such training were also saying. His insistence that 'political interference' was the cause of all health problems implied that decision-making by elected officials has no place in a democracy. He failed to say why most citizens of a country which had endured racial minority rule should now want to be governed, on health issues, by a minority composed of scientists who ignored the daily news. He also, of course, repeated the fallacy that there was a single 'science' on Covid-19 (or many other issues) which was his and his fellow medical professionals' sole possession.

His account of how the virus should be fought and what the government should have done was incoherent. He was quoted as saying that the government should introduce a 'gradual' lockdown but also that it should simply have stopped mass gatherings. What is a 'gradual' lockdown? If the only proposed measure was a ban on gatherings, in what way was that a lockdown, gradual or not? His rationale that the poor had no means to store food is puzzling. Since food stores were open throughout the lockdown, why would they need to store it? Why was it a mistake to close schools, given the possibility that pupils might spread the virus? If the claim that lockdown wasn't really about readying the health system, what was it about? And why did most scientists who attacked the lockdown agree that it was needed initially?

These two medical scientists are singled out because they gave rather fuller explanations than, say, Mendelson, who simply insisted (at least in his reported utterances) that the restrictions end because mass infection was inevitable, without saying why, just as he did not justify his claim that three in five people were doomed to be infected. Ironically, as will be seen, the evidence suggests that he had the equation precisely the wrong way around. It was not that the lockdown needed to go because many cases were inevitable, but that many cases were inevitable because too little was done to protect public health. In sum, it is difficult to escape the conclusion that the anti-lockdown chorus was expressing a general suburban sentiment presented as a scientific position.

A significant feature of the episode was the instant reaction of academics and journalists who cover Covid-19. They elevated Gray into a fighter for freedom who was being persecuted by an irrational and authoritarian government. Mkhize's response objected not to her right to speak but to her tone and the fact that she had not raised the issue with the department. Gray did not challenge the minister's assertion that her advice had not been ignored because she had never offered it. He did not threaten any action against her. Academic freedom does not, as many in the South African debate assume, mean the right not to be criticised. Would the university vice-chancellor who signed the statement supporting her have been similarly well disposed to academics at his university who attacked him in intemperate terms? We know the answer – in a much-discussed book, Habib angrily responded to his academic colleagues who challenged the university's approach to protest under his leadership in terms which made the minister's response seem mild by comparison.[28] So, if vice-chancellors reply angrily to their critics, academic freedom is preserved. If ministers do this in a milder tone, it is violated.

It would have been odd if the minister had not responded, given that the source of the attack headed an important official research council which had a working relationship with his department. Since Gray had dismissed the government's response using particularly insulting language, his response was measured and moderate. Pillay's call to investigate her could be seen as threatening and did seem to show that he lacked the political skills of his minister, but no investigation was ever launched. In any event, when the head of the country's leading medical research institution denounces the government in deeply insulting terms, asking it to find out what she had in mind ranks very, very low as a human rights abuse. But evidence was not a factor in the chorus of praise and support – Dasoo, Madhi and Mendelson have been portrayed as fearless challengers of power by the media and no one in authority has ever even bothered to issue a statement criticising them, let alone threatened action against them. Not one of the claims by scientists discussed here – or indeed anything else which they said – was ever challenged by the media. They were never asked to justify their position. Gray's claim about malnutrition at Baragwanath, which would have undermined the credibility of a medical intern, was simply noted as an error before the adoration resumed. Had a government minister made the same statement, they would have faced sustained questioning and unabated ridicule.

This incident says far more about South Africa's divisions and the public debate which reflects them than about the merits or demerits of lockdowns. This is hardly the first time that a government critic has been treated as a martyr to free expression despite the fact that their 'punishment' consisted of a reply from someone in the government. The same treatment was afforded a business leader who called government leaders a 'strange breed' and implied that they were morally or intellectually defective and a major bank which flighted an ad in which a student urged voters to reject the government. Both were forced to endure nothing worse than replies from the government yet both were portrayed as victims of gross human rights abuses.[29]

This reflected the dynamics within 'First World' South Africa mentioned in chapter 1 – the government is assumed to represent the 'Third World' even though it does not and so it is automatically assumed to be the problem unless the contrary is proven (and sometimes even then). Businesspeople and professionals are, by contrast, impeccable examples of 'First World' excellence and are thus the solution unless the contrary is proven (and sometimes even then). Medical scientists fall into this latter category. A representative of the 'First World' who attacks the government is automatically assumed to have the right to say whatever they like and the government is denounced if it does so much as reply. The scientists were lionised and the government denounced not because the superior logic of the former won the argument, or because the government tried to silence them, but because they were exemplars of a 'First World' forced to endure the depredations of a government which was voted for by the 'Third World', even though it was no more sensitive to its concerns than the rest of the 'First World'.

None of this means that the government's rules were always appropriate. Where, as Dasoo suggests, they relied on controlling people, they were not. Nor does it mean that opposition to a lockdown is automatically a sign of 'First World' prejudice. Lockdowns are only one of a variety of measures to fight a pandemic – Taiwan was able to prevent a severe epidemic without locking down.[30] But both the scientists' attack and the fact that they emerged as middle-class heroes were far more about how sections of the 'First World' see the country, and thus the fight against the pandemic, than the claimed clash between science and government. A charitable view is that the scientists and their allies so vividly remembered the HIV conflict that they saw it happening again even when it wasn't. But the similarity between this dynamic and that in countless other cases suggests that the core issue was who the 'First World' considered 'civilised' and 'sophisticated' and who it did not.

The dispute was also ironic because the antagonists were, in reality, on the same side. Karim often seemed to be as much the target of their ire as the minister and the government – hence, for example, the implication that Mkhize had chosen him over Gray because it wanted someone who agreed with it rather than a critic. His much-quoted April presentation contained a slide which suggested that the lockdown should remain in force if case numbers were high,[31] which seemed of no interest to the other scientists. But in the same presentation and in a later interview, he endorsed the consensus that many cases and deaths were inevitable. In late November, in response to questions about a second wave of infections, he said that the country was 'in a good position of low transmission' outside the Eastern Cape and the Garden Route area of the Western Cape, where infections were growing sharply.[32] In the Introduction, it was noted that, at the time he spoke, some 1 600 new cases a day had been identified since August, many times higher than the number of daily cases which prompted some other countries to take strong protective measures. In Karim's view, a daily case rate which would have caused alarm from Seoul to Kigali was 'a good position of low transmission'.

The government view, too, was not fundamentally at odds with that of its critics. It did, of course, impose restrictions they disliked, although these were not the arbitrary flights of fancy of which Gray complained. It was noted earlier that they stemmed from the belief, widespread in 'First World' South Africa, that the townships and shack settlements were incapable of protecting themselves and so needed to be forced. But, in March, before the first lockdown was imposed, Mkhize said that 'in our estimation', '60 to 70% will be affected by the virus in our communities. We cannot hide that.' He added that 'it does not mean it will be a severe disease to all of us, it will be severe to … 20%.'[33] It is not clear from the report whether he meant that this proportion of the population would be infected or whether they would merely be 'affected', which would presumably mean that a family member or someone important to them would contract the virus. The 20 per cent seems to be a proportion of those infected, not the population, since he urged the country to 'make sure that at every time the 20% is small',[34] in other words, that there were less cases and so less people with severe disease at any one time. But this is, nevertheless, a dire prediction.

The minister's expectation meant, assuming a population of some 60 million, that at least 40 million would fall ill and around eight million would contract a 'severe case'. Even if he meant only affected and we assume, say, that each ill person would affect the lives of eight others, that still meant five million cases and a million gravely ill people. At the very least, he expected significantly more people to become severely ill than the total number of cases reported by end November. If we assume a case fatality rate – the number of people testing positive who lose their lives – of slightly more than two per cent, around the global average, he expected anything from at least 100 000 to 800 000 deaths (the first figure is based on five million cases, the second on 40 million). However we interpret the minister's warning, he expected many people to fall very ill and many to die.

Why, if this was inevitable, did he urge the country to keep cases as low as possible? The answer is not entirely clear because the government's message was unclear throughout. On the one hand, as Mkhize's comments show, it signalled that there was little or nothing it could do about Covid-19. On the other, particularly in the initial phases, it seemed to be imbued with what James Scott calls 'high modernism', the belief that governments can use 'scientific laws' to force society to do anything that they want it to do.[35] As this author pointed out in May:

> A comment by Minister of Trade and Industry Ebrahim Patel shows where the bizarre official mixture of fatalism, which assumes that disaster is inevitable, and a belief that the government has supernatural powers, can lead. Official projections first said the epidemic would peak in June or July ... Patel told a briefing that, because mid-year was the flu season, the government had decided to postpone the peak to September. So, the virus is so powerful that we cannot stop it, but it can also be made to delay its peak on the orders of the revealingly named National Coronavirus Command Council.[36]

The government never said precisely why it was urging people to avoid what it claimed to be inevitable. But it, too, believed that 'getting the health system ready' was key to fighting the virus. In an address to the nation on 24 May, Ramaphosa said,

> As a result of the measures we imposed – and the sacrifices you made – we have managed to slow the rate of infection and prevent our health facilities from being overwhelmed. We have used the time during the lockdown to build up an extensive public health

response and prepare our health system for the anticipated surge in infections.[37]

The goal of delaying the inevitable was, therefore, to ensure that the health system could cope with infections, a view entirely compatible with that of those scientists who went beyond simply denouncing lockdowns to suggesting something even approaching a credible alternative. The two sides may have disagreed on the extent of the inconvenience which should be imposed on the suburbs to ensure that the health system could cope (regardless of whether it could help patients) but they agreed that a severe epidemic was inevitable. This was no abstract point. It presumably lay at the heart of the easing of restrictions in circumstances which had far more to do with the lobbying of interest groups than with the 'carefully calibrated' science which the government claimed lay at the heart of its approach.

THE SUBURBS ON THE MARCH

In late March, when the government announced the beginning of the lockdown, Ramaphosa and some of his ministers appeared in front of the cameras with representatives of Business for South Africa, an initiative launched by organised business associations. The business representatives pledged support for the fight against the virus and offered support programmes, including the provision of ventilators and personal protective equipment. In mid-April, the organisation announced its support for an extension of the lockdown beyond 16 April.[38]

Photographs of the two delegations suggest that, despite the agreement to work together, there was a degree of awkwardness between them. The relationship between business and government is another of those 'First World' dynamics discussed in chapter 1 in which tension blends with mutual interest. The two have little option but to work together on issues which affect the health of the market economy. From the time South African industrialisation began, they have been obliged to cooperate even when they are publicly at odds.[39] But that does not mean the relationship is inherently friendly.

For much of the life of apartheid, business and the political leadership of the black majority were on opposite sides of the fence. While sections of business opposed some of the minority government's racial policies, many businesspeople harboured racial attitudes not unlike those of the state leadership. Most above a particular size did business with the government, even though their senior executives criticised its policy. This prompted many in what was to become the ANC government to conclude that private business was irrevocably opposed to black interests. While these attitudes eroded as they were absorbed into 'First World' South Africa, lingering suspicions remain. Key corporations made their peace with the ANC in the late 1980s but many in business share the view that the governing party is incompetent and hostile to business, a view assiduously encouraged by the financial media. This deepens the lack of trust on both sides. Ramaphosa's presidency has brought them closer together – he is a former businessman who feels at home with people in business. But it has not entirely wiped clean the slate created by history. The relationship remains instrumental – both sides need to make use of the other – not a meeting of minds.

Given this, it seemed likely that businesses wanted something in return for patriotism, and so it quickly proved. As early as mid-April, when Business for South Africa diverged from the suburban consensus by backing the lockdown extension, it was already preparing to influence the government's response to the virus. Its website revealed that it had established an Economic Intervention work group, one of three such groups which were meant to shape its contribution. It offered a list of its areas of interest; many seemed designed to ensure a more effective and just response. This included assistance on a project which aimed to acquire ventilators, a call on corporate members to assist small and medium enterprises by paying them by 20 April, monitoring 'price gouging' and suggesting measures to 'reduce predatory pricing'. But most of the other focuses seemed to be leading in a particular direction. They included a macroeconomic analysis which would 'suggest a range of support and relief packages'; 'critical inputs provided to government to expand the definition of essential goods and services'; influencing changes to rules 'that opened up port capacity and the movement of essential cargo from the ports'; providing 'supporting interventions for SMMEs [small, medium and micro enterprises], formal and informal'; and 'facilitating exemptions for international flights and air crew to expedite the receipt of essential air cargo, particularly medical supplies.'[40]

All of these could play a role in urging a lifting of restrictions. One support package recommended by the macroeconomic analysis might be the lifting of controls; expanding 'essential goods and services' could mean opening up more activities, while the focus on opening ports and exemptions for flights was self-explanatory. The support intervention for small and medium enterprises could include lobbying to reopen them. This does not mean that the offer of help was simply a ploy to win the government over – fighting Covid-19 was in business's interest. But it did mean that Business for South Africa was not simply a vehicle to enable business to help fight the virus, as it was frequently portrayed. It was also a lobby, and a well-resourced one at that. It soon began to wield that influence to push the government to lift restrictions to open up the economy.

Organised business began to lobby openly for the removal of restrictions from the beginning of May. But the financial media – which often takes its cue from sources in business – and some economists began their campaign for opening up immediately after the lockdown was extended beyond 16 April. On 19 April, a financial publication reported that 'South Africans' had assumed that all restrictions would end on 16 April when they 'would again be allowed to move around freely, go to a restaurant, drive to work, or stop in at the corner café to pick up a packet of cigarettes. Businesses would reopen and factories start up. But on Friday the country was still in lockdown.' It quoted an economist calling for the economy to be reopened (but did, in fairness, point out also that a food conglomerate had been forced to close one of its bakeries after administrative staff tested positive for Covid-19).[41] It seemed fair to assume that the 'South Africans' in question were those who lived in suburbs and were active in business.

The article may have been the first of its kind but was hardly the last. From mid-April, the financial media began pressing for reopening the economy. They were soon joined by the rest of the media, which began fixating on the plight of businesses which could not operate in the lockdown. Quickly, the businesses realised that they could expect a sympathetic platform and began approaching the media with their accounts of distress. In contrast to some other countries, this was never balanced by pictures of the reality in hospitals, where the suffering which Covid-19 brought offered a more harrowing picture than that which businesses were able to paint of their own distress.

The lobby entered the public domain on 6 May, when Business for South Africa called for 'an urgent reopening of the economy'. It said it was 'forcefully' engaging with the government on level 4 regulations, advocating strongly, for instance, 'for all e-commerce to be reopened'. Stavros Nicolaou, head of the group's health workstream (he is an executive in a pharmaceutical company), said the objective of the lockdown had been to prepare the health services for what lay ahead. 'We are certainly in a better position now than we were to save lives,' he said.[42] The lobby was soon joined by Business Unity South Africa, whose chief executive Cas Coovadia said in mid-May that there was 'a greater appreciation in the government of the economic costs of SA's national lockdown and acceptance that the way it's being implemented has limited value in mitigating health risks'. Lest there be any doubt about which side the publication which quoted him was on, its report of his remarks was headlined 'Government May be Seeing the Light on Need to Open Economy',[43] which implied that the issue was so cut and dried that the government was simply being urged to do what was patently rational.

This chorus ignored the human toll wrought by Covid-19, but it also paid no heed to evidence that the obstacle to economic recovery was the virus, not the measures which protected against it, which meant that restrictions which damaged the economy in the short term would restore it to health quicker if they eliminated the virus.[44] This was the view not of tree-hugging socialists but some very mainstream economists, including the International Monetary Fund (IMF) which observed in October that 'although easing lockdowns can lead to a partial recovery, economic activity is likely to remain subdued until health risks abate.'[45] Instead, it took refuge in cliché: it became common for commentators to insist that the response to the virus was a choice between 'lives' and 'livelihoods'. This denied the possibility that saving lives might be the only way to save livelihoods. The occasional attempt to challenge this view was, to the extent that it was recognised at all, given a polite but brief hearing and then dismissed from view. If we recall that the national debate is the territory of insiders alone, it was not uncharitable to assume that this response had something to do with the fact that the insiders did not feel that their lives were under threat but feared that their livelihoods might be diminished.

From the middle of April, the government faced a sustained lobby to open the economy which enjoyed the full support of all the media – 'First World' South Africa united to show its suspected 'Third World' government that its interests lay with them. Since it was itself very much part of the 'First World', the government began to 'see the light' on many of these issues and regulations were repeatedly eased until September, when lockdown level 1 was introduced, reducing the restrictions to not much more than a ban on mass gatherings.[46] By this time, restaurants and some other forms of entertainment, usually seen as high risks in a pandemic, were also opened.

While business's concerns were given priority, another lobby which wielded influence was religious leaders. In May, around the same time as organised business was pressing for a reopening, they were doing the same. On 21 May, it was reported that Ramaphosa had 'received an overwhelming request from religious leaders to open places of worship when government drops the Covid-19 lockdown to Level 3.'[47] They did not have to wait long – days later, the government announced that it would indeed allow places of worship to open albeit 'with strict conditions in place.'[48] While not all religious leaders were eager to open and some publicly announced that they would not, the demand to allow services enjoyed broad support among leadership in all the country's faiths. This was another sharp contrast with the rest of the continent, where 'faith-based organisations have been vital in creating awareness about Covid-19, addressing gender-based violence, and countering coronavirus misinformation.'[49]

Sport plays an important role in South Africa, so it was predictable that it, too, would give the media new opportunities to portray the government as a heartless trampler on the well-being of the wealthier classes. In late April, the country confronted the sombre warning that a third of its golf clubs might not survive the lockdown but was also assured that 'bodies are now lobbying hard to get golf courses open again during the more relaxed versions of lockup [sic], even though organised sport is very low on the list of priority sectors.'[50] Sport had a little longer to wait than religion, but by July it too had its way and all 'elite' or professional contact sports (and amateur sport which did not require contact) were allowed, albeit without spectators. At the same time, 'cinemas, theatres, museums, libraries and galleries' were opened although only a maximum of 50 people were allowed to attend,[51] but not before a decision that only professional contact sport would be allowed (rather than its amateur equivalent) was said to have 'pushed the sporting industry closer to the brink of collapse.'[52]

In the presentation to the WHO cited earlier, Mkhize warned, in a slide titled 'Lessons Learned', that 'there are serious risks associated with lifting lockdown restrictions too soon.'[53] It is not clear whether this was an admission that the lobbies had pushed the government too far too soon. But, if it was not, it should have been. The only risk of importance to the 'risk adjusted strategy' seemed to be the risk of upsetting interest groups. While a sustained 'hard' lockdown was never a possibility and may, in any event, not have been necessary, it is hard to believe that the decisions to open up in the face of lobbying were about 'following the science', not negotiating the shoals of South Africa's interest group politics.

WHOSE SCIENCE?

From the time that the lockdown was renewed in mid-April, a sustained lobby by interest groups, most notably business, prompted a phased relaxation of regulations which endured until the last days of 2020, when the 'second wave' of infections prompted a return to a modified level 3. Religious services were again not permitted and alcohol sales were again banned but business activity, including restaurants, was allowed.[54]

If the medical scientists who denounced the lockdown were right, this was presumably a triumph for science – Gray and Dasoo had, after all, insisted that restrictions were unscientific and Madhi and Mendelson clearly agreed even if they used less direct language. But, whether or not the changes were necessary, they ignored international scientific common sense and the science which was embraced at the outset of the pandemic. On the first score, South Africa's response required it to lift restrictions even as case numbers were rising. This was certainly not unique – many states in the USA did the same, as did much of Latin America.⁵⁵ But it does not require training in medical science to work out that allowing freedom of movement will increase cases. The countries and regions which have adopted this approach have experienced far more severe waves of cases and deaths than those which eased restrictions only when case numbers and deaths began to fall.

Two very different realities enabled countries to ease restrictions only when case numbers fell. The countries which kept cases and deaths down to very low levels tended to restrict early and reopen when they had suppressed cases. East Asia and New Zealand are much-quoted examples; they could emerge from restrictions because they had contained the virus. The other, far more familiar to the South African debate, is that countries in Western Europe and some states in the USA which locked down late, when case numbers were high, were able to relax restrictions when they succeeded in driving infection numbers down (although the relaxation came with a huge cost when the 'second wave' engulfed them). It is hard to see how easing restrictions as cases increase could contribute to the Holy Grail of protecting the health system – or how it could make the virus any easier to contain.

Nor was this pattern consistent with Karim's approach, despite his insistence that the virus could not be stopped. In his April presentation, he had, as noted earlier, spelled out what he called the epidemiological view of when restrictions would be eased. After 16 April, the lockdown should be extended if there were more than 90 cases per day, while 'daily increases of between 45 and 89 may open the door to an easing of restrictions.'⁵⁶ While he was talking specifically about whether the lockdown should be extended on 16 April, it is hard to see why this criterion should not apply to the easing of restrictions in general. The government's response to the lobbies entirely ignored this advice. Contrary to Gray's claim (and that of her colleagues), it is the call to ease the restrictions which was unscientific (whether it was 'nonsensical' was in the eye of the beholder).

On 1 May, the country moved to lockdown level 4 which slightly eased the restrictions on leaving homes and allowed some businesses to reopen subject to restrictions designed to curb the spread of the virus.[57] Ramaphosa announced the change on 23 April. But, in the days before he did, cases were rising on average by 192 a day, more than double the number which, according to Karim, should force a continued lockdown.[58] On 24 May, Ramaphosa announced that the country would move to lockdown level 3 from 1 June. This meant that alcohol sales were permitted for part of the week and most business sectors (excluding hospitality) would reopen (although tobacco sales were still banned). Business travel was also allowed albeit with restrictions,[59] controls on taking exercise were further relaxed and religious services resumed. In the month before this announcement, cases had risen by more than 600 a day,[60] well over six times the number which Karim said was needed to maintain the restrictions. The decision to open cinemas and other indoor activities such as museums and galleries was taken when cases had been rising by, on average, 5 585 a day over the previous month.[61]

Two points about this pattern stand out. First, none of the decisions to ease restrictions were remotely consistent with Karim's criteria. It is hard to see in any of this a carefully calibrated 'risk adjusted strategy' which 'followed the science' – unless the science is assumed to be the sweeping statements medical scientists make in media interviews. Decisions were determined by the power and influence of lobbies. This was a political and social process, not one based on the findings of laboratory experiments. That is not necessarily a criticism; government is political and social and 'the science' was contested. But it does expose the conceit of claiming that political and social processes are 'scientific'. It was probably inevitable that Karim's version of 'the science' wilted under the scorn of 'First World' South Africa. But whatever was followed, it was not 'the science'. Second, each decision to lift restrictions was followed by an increase in infections. This was presumably expected by scientists since it was consistent with a view which insisted that many cases and deaths were inevitable. But it needs stressing because the dominant view also claims that the lockdown did nothing to stem cases and deaths.

The evidence suggests otherwise. Karim's celebrated mid-April presentation had marvelled at the degree to which, in his view, South Africa's case and deaths trajectory was unexpectedly low. So impressed was he that he claimed that 'SA's epidemic trajectory is unique.'[62] It wasn't, of course – it was 'unique' only when compared to the USA and Western Europe. But he also pointed out that cases were rising 'exponentially' when the virus arrived, making the trend even more remarkable. The only plausible explanation was the effect of the lockdown. This was further confirmed by a tracking exercise conducted by Trade and Industry Policy Strategies, a research organisation which offered detailed data on case and fatality trends.[63] Its numbers show that, until the move to level 3, only the Western Cape and, to a lesser extent, the Eastern Cape experienced high increases in case numbers (discussed further in chapter 4). In seven provinces, including the country's economic hub, Gauteng, case numbers and deaths did follow the pattern which excited Karim.

Not every decision to lift regulations increased the spread of the virus. But some clearly did – allowing business travel as case numbers soar seems particularly hard to defend, especially since the travellers presumably all could comfortably work remotely. Nor was there a clear rationale for allowing people to congregate in restaurants and, later, bars where the potential for spreading the virus seems great. The restrictions did protect life and health. This does not mean that they were sustainable indefinitely or even for a lengthy period. But the lobby to remove them began after three weeks, not three months, which makes it even harder to square with 'following the science'.

Why did this happen? The anti-lockdown lobbies insisted that 'South Africans' could not bear the restrictions any longer. It is a stock feature of the country's 'First World' debate that the 'Third World' majority is spoken about and for but never speaks. More specifically, it is common to insist that any policy preference, even those which are patently designed to protect the interests of those who have more than enough, is really meant to assist 'the poor'. But here, as in many of the other cases, what evidence we have suggests that many South Africans were not only comfortable with the measures but may well have preferred stricter curbs than the government was willing to introduce.

It was mentioned earlier that township residents were stubbornly more concerned about staying out of hospital and alive than American researchers felt they should be. So was the palpable fear of travelling in taxis, a concern to which the government merely paid lip service. It is open to question whether anyone could be safe from the virus in a 70 per cent full minibus. However, the point was moot because the drivers – whose margins are low, making it essential to transport as many people as possible as swiftly as possible – filled their vehicles and ignored rules requiring passengers to be distanced from each other and windows to be open to allow ventilation, despite the fact that law enforcement officials were on hand who were meant to prevent this.[64] The minister of transport, Fikile Mbalula, responded with loud indignation but there was no evidence that anything changed because he was angry.[65] The taxi industry is a powerful lobby – far more powerful than 'the science' (since restricting taxis was one protective measure which the medical scientists advised).

Further evidence is offered by a controversy over schools. Opening schools is a favourite of anti-lockdown lobbies everywhere. The stated rationale is the interests of pupils but the fact that this makes it easier for parents to return to work may also play a role. The closure of schools was one of the many targets of Gray's anger. But teacher unions and, more important for this argument, many parents were opposed to opening schools in the midst of a pandemic. Mahlamola Kekana, president of the National Association of Parents in School

Governance, said in an affidavit opposing the attempt by the official opposition, the DA, to persuade courts to overturn the lockdown regulations, that 'millions' of parents opposed reopening schools unless they demonstrated clearly they were equipped to protect teachers and learners. Kekana described 'the blanket one-size-fits-all national re-opening of schools' as 'patently irrational and arbitrary'.[66] While interest associations often exaggerate their support, and there is no doubt an added incentive to this in an attempt to convince a court, a survey by the University of Johannesburg and the Human Sciences Research Council (HSRC), conducted between 30 December 2020 and 6 January 2021, supported Kekana's claim. It found that 53 per cent of adults were opposed to reopening schools as scheduled because the country was then experiencing the 'second wave' of infections. A further 19 per cent wanted only grades 7 and 12 (the finishing years for primary and high school) to reopen, making a 72 per cent majority in favour of restrictions. The survey also found a significant racial divide in attitudes to opening schools: among whites, only 37 per cent opposed reopening, while majorities were reported among everyone else.[67]

So, whether you believed that restrictions were 'unscientific and nonsensical' or that lifting them was 'arbitrary and irrational' depended on your position in society, not scientific training. If the survey is accurate, the majority of whites agree with Gray, the majority of the rest of the country with Kekana and the teachers' trade unions. Which view expressed the science? Not surprisingly, given that there is no scientific consensus on Covid-19, both and neither – there was no agreement on whether schools should reopen or on how to protect learners and teachers when they were.[68] So at issue was not who knew the science and who did not but differing interests and perspectives, products of where people sit in society. 'The suburbs' is not simply a euphemism for 'white' – many black people have moved to suburbs. But, since only a tiny handful of whites don't live in suburbs and the majority of blacks live in townships (including, of course, those established to house the black racial minorities, 'coloured' and Indian people), it does not seem unreasonable to argue that the pressure to open restrictions came primarily from the suburbs. There is also suggestive evidence, presented here, that majority opinion in townships and shack settlements may well have supported restrictions (or at least some of them) which the suburbs opposed or to which they were indifferent.

The government, then, did not 'follow the science'. It followed the suburbs, even if it parted company with them for a while. It did this not only because most people in government, public servants as well as elected politicians, live in suburbs but because crucial to the life of the suburbs, understood as a metaphor for 'First World' South Africa, was the existence of strongly organised and influential lobbies that could rely on loud and sustained media support for their campaign to ensure that the rules did not prevent them from conducting the activities to which they considered themselves entitled. The fact that the scientists, or at least those who hogged the headlines, insisted (despite the reservations of some about taxis and public gatherings) that restrictions were a problem, says more about the influence of 'First World' thinking in South Africa on those who live in suburbs, including medical scientists, than about their research.

The lesson of the anti-lockdown lobby's success in persuading the government to roll back restrictions is not that an undisputed scientific view of what was needed was ignored. Rather, what unravelled was the claim that the government was 'following the science'. The response to Covid-19 suggests that 'following the science' may always have been code for 'listening to the suburbs'. Chapter 4 will expand on this but 'the science' as it was understood in South Africa was, in reality, the expression of a particular 'First World' perspective which is deeply sceptical of the ability of majority-ruled governments to effectively fight pandemics (or do much else), which assumes that most

South Africans are incapable of protecting themselves and that the economic, cultural and leisure priorities of the suburbs take precedence unless the suburbs feel themselves threatened.

The influence of lobbies is hardly a uniquely South African reality. It is a standard feature of all societies.[69] But the (often successful) lobby against restrictions was different to similar processes in the rest of the continent. Other African governments are lobbied by professional and business associations.[70] They also face popular protest – on Covid-19 regulations as well as other issues.[71] But the lobbies cannot rely on the support of a significant sector of the citizenry; the protestors are not represented in the corridors of power. In South Africa, the meetings with business organisations and religious leaders were only a part of the pressure for the lifting of restrictions. Their efforts – and particularly those of business – were supported by media which repeatedly stressed the damage done to businesses while the harm done by the disease was largely reduced to a daily recitation of official case fatality – and, of course, recovery – figures. Opposition political parties, citizens' organisations and individuals using digital media added to the chorus. This quickly created a climate of opinion among the minority who enjoyed access to the debate which painted the fight against the virus as the problem, not the virus itself.

At play was not the 'interest group politics' so beloved of some political scientists. The government rarely faced multiple voices, some demanding that the rules go, others insisting that they stay. There was little lively debate and contest for influence between contending interests. With one exception – the opposition of teachers' unions and parent associations to reopening schools – only one voice was heard, that which wanted the restrictions eased or ended. This offers an added dimension to the influence of the medical scientists. When they lobbied against the lockdown, they began with an advantage in a country where those who are heard assume that government is a site of incompetence and impure motives; anything in the suburbs outside the government, particular businesses and professionals (such as scientists) a hub of probity and ability. They were feted because their voices augmented a chorus willing to venerate anyone who launched an attack on the restrictions. The government faced not a lobby but a loud consensus in 'First World' society which could be conveyed by a variety of institutions and organisations all saying the same thing. No other African country faced anything remotely similar.

The government might have dug in despite this if it was, as the 'First World' thought, really the voice of the 'Third World'. But it wasn't. Despite the loud arguments about the sale of cigarettes or alcohol (and in both cases the restrictions enjoyed significant support within the 'First World'[72]), and repeated attempts in the media and by the industries fighting restrictions to portray it as authoritarian, left-wing and incompetent (some responses literally did see the restrictions as a communist plot[73]), they inhabited the same world. The government was not bullied or browbeaten into removing the restrictions. It did so because the language of the lobby made sense to it. And this in turn assured that the country's response to Covid-19 reflected not what 'the science' said, but what 'First World' South Africa wanted.

CHAPTER
4

The Blank Cheque

One of democracy's core functions is to hold power accountable. 'Mainstream development orthodoxy' also tells us that accountability is essential to ensuring that government serves everyone, including people living in poverty.[1]

In most conventional accounts, that usually means holding the government accountable. Because citizens enjoy rights, they are able to speak, organise and act in concert to ensure that those who govern tell them what they are doing and why they are doing it. If what they are doing is not what citizens want, they face vocal pressure to change.[2] But, contrary to the claims of devotees of the unfettered market, accountability is not restricted to government – it can equally well be demanded of private interests whose actions and decisions affect the lives and interests of the citizenry.

Accountability is rarely a product of the efforts of individuals. It stems from institutions and organisations and how groups use them. The media (digital as well as conventional), the academy and citizens' organisations enable the people to demand answers and to insist on change if they do not like what they hear. This should ensure government that is more responsive to the needs of citizens. While the real world of democracy is much messier than this account suggests, accountability understood in this way has, across the globe, forced the holders of power to accommodate the needs and wishes of citizens. There can be few issues on which this is more needed than a country's response to a pandemic which threatens the health and well-being of everyone who lives within its borders. Democracies should be better equipped to deal with pandemics than authoritarian societies because those who decide how to respond are more likely to be forced to explain and to correct behaviours and policies which do not meet citizens' needs. But accountability is more complicated than that.

Democratic rights make accountability possible but they do not make it inevitable unless people can and will use them to hold power to account. Not all citizens enjoy the same power to hold government to account. Citizens who have a pressing interest in making themselves heard are often powerless and so the accountability relationship simply does not work for them. A consequence of the realities discussed in chapter 1 is that, in South Africa, it is the 'insiders' who join the organisations and make use of the institutions which hold power holders to account.[3] Accountability will only be demanded if the issue on which power holders need to account is of concern to those who are able to demand it.

Only one of South Africa's power holders seemed to be held to account for its response to the pandemic – the government. The scientists received not a single critical question. The business or religious lobbies who were vocal on the damage wrought by restrictions but muted on the harm the pandemic has done to tens of thousands of families were not challenged. The media which, besides fawning over scientists and business lobbies alike, offered little coherent information on the pandemic beyond reporting official statistics and statements, often in a way which showed that they had failed to understand them, was never criticised.

But has the government really been held to account? The pressure it faced focused purely on the restrictions it imposed. This became all-consuming, the only issue which received public attention. So pervasive did it become that any attempt to discuss the more fundamental issue, whether it was doing as much as it could to prevent people falling ill and dying, was drowned out by demands that whoever was trying to do this declare themselves for or against 'the lockdown'. And yet it was the issue which was brushed aside which cried out for demands for accountability. On this, the government and anyone else responsible for responding to Covid-19 was given a blank cheque. We will never know how many illnesses and deaths could have been avoided if the government and the other power holders had faced pressure to curb them. But it does seem reasonable to expect that Covid-19 would have done less damage if that had happened.

The power holders had a blank cheque not because those who are able to hold power to account were ill-informed, lazy or unable to concentrate – it is common in the South African debate to reduce deep-rooted realities to the flaws of individuals. This misunderstands most issues, and it would certainly fail to grasp why the power holders were never held to account for the way they approached the task of keeping people alive and healthy. The debate had little interest in demanding measures to protect people because, during 2020, the burden of Covid-19 fell predominantly on the townships and shack settlements. This is not to say that no one in the suburbs contracted the virus or lost their lives to it. But, because the overwhelming majority of those who did suffer were in the 'Third World', the debate remained far more worried about the measures used to respond to the virus than the virus itself.

Usually, those who enjoy access to the debate pay no price for ignoring the needs and concerns of South Africa's 'Third World'. Chapter 1 showed that the life experiences of the two worlds differ so much that the costs to the minority of ignoring the reality of the majority are slight. The 'First World' can, therefore, largely ignore the experience of the 'Third', even when they have consequences for the well-being of the suburbs. Crime may well be a suburban consequence of neglecting 'Third World' realities but the link is rarely made in the 'First World' – the life circumstances of the perpetrators are of no interest to the debate. Economic exclusion suppresses growth by reducing the pool of people able to contribute to it and limiting domestic consumer markets. It may strain the financial system or labour bargaining as people borrow beyond their means to pay for consumer goods[4] or demand large wage increases to feed unemployed family members.[5] But again the connection is not made and, given the biases of the 'First World', this is likely to be blamed on 'financial illiteracy'[6] or 'union greed'.[7]

In this case, the failure (or unwillingness) to suppress infections during much of 2020 ensured not only a 'second wave' but the emergence of a new, more transmissible, strain of the virus which did affect the suburbs more severely, ensuring that there was more pressure on private than public hospitals.[8] But not even this prompted pressure on the authorities to explain why they were not stemming case numbers – by then, vaccines had been developed. Since these were products of medical technology and, therefore, of curative medicine, they were seized upon as a solution[9] and rising case numbers were blamed on the government's failure to buy them. Beyond that, and probably because the 'second wave' did not last long, the rising case numbers were treated as unavoidable and no one was held to account for them.

FAILING THE TEST

Inevitably, the lack of accountability ensured that flaws in the response to the virus were barely noticed and never challenged. The loud voices, sweeping statements and derision with which 'First World' South

Africa reacted to the lockdown were never employed to ask why so many people were falling ill and dying.

The prime example was the failure of testing and tracing. The great 'debate' discussed in chapter 3 was so fixated on the restrictions imposed during lockdown that there was no discussion on why they were needed in the first place. No one believes that lockdowns could, on their own, defeat viruses. At best they can reduce case numbers dramatically but not entirely. They have a limited lifespan since, of course, economies cannot be suspended for long. Even in China, where the authorities, who do not need to burden themselves with democratic niceties, could and did at times lock down cities for long periods, it was not these restrictions alone which suppressed the virus.

The purpose of lockdowns is, rather, to drive down case numbers. But, if the solution is to have lasting benefits, the goal is not to 'ready the health system' but to ensure that numbers are so low that it becomes possible to test infected people, trace their contacts, and ensure that both are isolated so that the virus cannot spread. Besides its fixation with the health system, South Africa's response did include testing and tracing – chapter 2 noted Karim's remarks on the community health workers who were meant to identify cases.

Despite this, testing and tracing failed – the country would not have been easing restrictions amid rising infections had it succeeded. In this Madhi and Mendelson were correct, despite their strange fatalism which questioned the benefits of tracing. It is not clear what role community health workers played as no one followed up on Karim's announcement by asking what they were doing and how they helped to protect people. Testing became the subject of public discussion as the government published figures on how many millions had been tested[10] but not because the debate cared whether it protected anyone. Tests became another marker of the divide between 'First World' and the rest, a sign of 'sophistication' and modernity.

The fact that high numbers were recorded in the Western Cape during the strict lockdown prompted a response which shows how events in South Africa were a microcosm of those across the globe. The province is arguably the capital of 'First World' South Africa. White and coloured people are in the majority (the result of an apartheid policy which used stricter influx control to ensure that these two groups were not outnumbered).[11] It is governed by the DA and is, for many in the suburbs, what a province should be. That it became the epicentre of infections meant much the same as the fact that the USA and UK experienced far worse epidemics than virtually all other countries – a challenge to 'First World' claims to superiority. ANC supporters saw an opportunity to challenge the DA's claim to govern more efficiently; since this was often code in the public mind for the claim that whites could govern better than blacks, the Western Cape's high numbers ignited racial dynamics too. White South Africa in particular felt the need to defend the honour of a province which was assumed to represent them, although whites are a minority in this province too.

Predictably, the stock response was that it had higher case numbers because it tested more. Trump made the same claim about the USA. In tones which brooked no disagreement, doubters were told that the Western Cape's high numbers were a sign of modernity and sophistication, not incompetence. But, in the Western Cape as in the US, this held no water. Hospital admissions and deaths were much higher than elsewhere which showed that testing was not the reason. Karim claimed it was an outbreak in shopping malls which was not controlled effectively.[12] In implied reply, others said epidemics in South Africa always started in the Western Cape because the province's openness to tourism made it more likely to experience high infection levels first. Some claims were much more exotic: altitude, ultraviolet rays and the weather were also claimed reasons.[13] The only explanation prohibited on this side of the debate was error by the provincial government. The debate remained unresolved – the divisiveness of the issue ensured that no serious attempt was made to discover why the province became the epicentre and it lost that status after some weeks. But the argument over the Western Cape showed that attitudes to testing were much the same as those to health systems identified by Alice Street.[14] They enabled higher numbers to be portrayed as a sign of superiority, not as evidence that the 'First World' might be fallible.

Also, testing on its own was of limited value unless it enabled the authorities to find contacts and prevent the virus spreading. This would happen only if positive tests were followed by quick contact tracing. A key reason for the testing programme's failure was that tests soon began to back up in the national laboratory.[15] The first politician to point this out may have been the Western Cape premier, Alan Winde, who wrote to Ramaphosa to complain about it.[16] It took days or even weeks for test results to return and this obviously made it impossible to find contacts quickly. This ensured that there was no effective tool to contain the virus. Infections would inevitably rise and the government would be forced either to ignore the wrath of the suburbs at huge economic cost or to relax restrictions while case numbers were growing. It is one of the great ironies of South Africa's battle against Covid-19 that the Achilles heel was not, as was widely assumed, people living in poverty in townships or shack settlements but a high-tech pathology lab.

Had test and trace worked, restrictions could have been lifted with little risk and the clichéd 'trade off' between lives and livelihoods would have been revealed for the misunderstanding it was. The great lockdown debate would have lost steam since restrictions would have been limited and their effect less obtrusive. Since so much was at stake, we would expect the blockages at the laboratory to trigger one of those familiar bouts of yelling at the government which are so common in the national debate, especially since the testing logjam was a worry to the provincial premier whom the debate was most likely to take seriously. But the pileup of tests at the laboratory was ignored by the debate. Parliament's select committee on health did address it in June when it discussed the laboratory's plans to address the problem[17] but this was not a response to public pressure and the hearings went unnoticed. They were held at least a month after the problem became evident, so much of the damage had already been done.

Madhi and Mendelson's article did mention the testing failure. But they did not raise their concerns when the problem emerged and they did not believe that an effective test and trace programme was possible. The voices which are often raised loudly to denounce government failure to do just about anything of concern to the insiders were silent. And so the feature of South Africa's democracy which is said to work best – the ability of a range of associations and institutions (such as the media) to hold the government to account – failed because it did not try to ensure that the lockdown at least gave the country a chance of suppressing the virus through a test and trace programme.

The government was also not held to account for tracing. As mentioned earlier, no one asked what the 28 000 community health workers mentioned by Karim were doing or how effective they were at discovering infected people. No one questioned why the government was not consulting African countries whose experience with Ebola had given them valuable lessons on how to trace contacts. The debate's fixation on curative medicine ensured no interest in tracing contacts. It does not believe South Africa could learn anything from the rest of the continent – certainly not on a health issue. In any event, since the fight against the pandemic was never seen by the debate as anything other than a strategy to 'ready the health system', tracing contacts to stop the spread was never considered important.

The failure to press the government on test and trace was the most glaring lapse in accountability in the crucial first phase of the pandemic. First responsibility for this rests with the medical scientists because it was they who shaped the debate's understanding of the virus. None of them stressed testing and tracing: Karim dealt with it in one slide of more than 20; Madhi and Mendelson, the only ones to see failed tracing as a problem, didn't believe an effective programme was possible anyway. None of the other scientists, so voluble in their campaign against the lockdown – and later so damning of the government when it did not buy vaccines once they were available – raised the issue. They were united in their belief that large numbers of cases and deaths were inevitable unless some form of curative medicine could be found to stop the virus. The 'First World' public agreed.

The media might have noticed international success stories and asked why the methods which were working elsewhere were not being applied here but they showed no inclination to find out anything which was not announced at government media conferences or contained in the presentations and webinars of the scientists. Nor did they show great interest in understanding how the virus worked. A radio anchor who thanked health workers for a drop in case numbers, entirely unaware that they treat people who are ill and have no role in preventing cases, may be extreme. But he is a symptom of the problem. Interviews with scientists are not only fawning – they rarely ask questions which might generate useful answers. Journalists fond of grilling ministers and officials didn't even seem to bother to prepare questions for scientists, who were assumed to know not only all the right answers but all the right questions too.

Even when the scientists were clearly wrong, they were celebrated, not interrogated. Besides the fact, mentioned in chapter 2, that it was not true that all countries were doomed to a severe epidemic – and the fact that no one seemed to mind Gray's lack of knowledge of malnutrition cases at public hospitals – no one held Madhi and Emeritus Professor Robin Wood to account when they doubted whether a 'second wave' would happen at all and added that, if it did, it would bring 'far fewer deaths'. Wood did qualify this by adding that 'any prediction that is made must be moderated with humility'; Madhi did not. The purpose of his prediction was, predictably, to support the ending of all restrictions except curbs on mass gatherings.[18] Neither was ever asked why his predictions were so wide of the mark since the 'second wave' was at least twice as deadly as the first.

Part of this could be explained by the state of the South African media. The industry is stressed and unable to cope with changing realities. At a time when new sources of news are supplanting their traditional role, they have reacted, in the main, not by offering higher-quality journalism but by retreating into 'opinion' which recycles the insider view of the world and whatever they are told by (private) authority figures. Specialist reporting, once common, is now rare – except for political and business reporting. There are few reporters who feel equipped to find out about health developments in other parts of the world and to ask the government and its scientists why they are not doing what others are doing well. There is no pressure for reporting which challenges conventional wisdom and much pressure against it. The contents of digital media are thus often used by South African media as a substitute for the real world: not much time or imagination are needed to turn tweets into a story. News coverage and analysis respond mainly to media conferences or claims or disputes on digital media.

These factors play a role but the media's failure to hold power to account has deeper roots. They are the voices of the 'First World'. The journalists are drawn from that world, they associate with others who inhabit it and they see the world through its eyes. We saw earlier how that ensured a grovelling deference to scientists; no criticism of the response to the virus would be taken seriously by the media unless the critics were scientists. This was demonstrated in early 2021, after vaccines were developed, when the scientists, not surprisingly given their addiction to medical technology, castigated the government for not buying them.[19] Again, they were free from critical questioning whatever they said.

The problem did not lie with the media alone. This is hardly surprising – the media industry is not a self-contained bubble, floating above society with its own interests and values. While it has problems of its own which explain poor quality, it is part of a network of institutions and organisations within the 'First World' milieu which interact with and often reinforce each other: political parties, business, the professions, the academy and citizens' organisations (or at least the type which are taken seriously in the debate). If any of these – particularly parties or businesses, which tend to attract more attention – had pressured the government to get test and trace or any other tool for combatting the crisis to work better, it would have faced huge pressure, not least because it takes the 'First World' far more seriously than the 'Third'. The media's failure was that of the 'First World'. One of democracy's core elements, holding power to account, did not operate because no one able to do this wanted to do it.

The initial support for the lockdown stemmed from a fear that everyone would be affected. To a degree everyone was. But, while the government did whatever it could to prevent data being used to determine the race or social and economic status of the people who died or took ill (presumably because it did not want groups with high infection rates to be labelled), the available evidence does show that townships were worst affected. The Gauteng Visual Analytics Platform, which breaks down 'hotspots' (suburbs with high case numbers), shows significantly more cases in townships than suburbs.[20] A study of blood donors by the National Blood Service found that black people were five times more likely to be affected than white people.[21] While the divide between the two worlds is not simply one between races, almost all whites live in suburbs and most blacks live in townships, so the finding does tell us something about the prevalence of the virus in the two 'worlds'. All visible politics in South Africa is insider politics, which in this context means 'First World' politics. The debate did not mind much that case and death numbers were rising, because the burden was borne mainly by others.

OTHER BLIND EYES

The same explanations apply to other failures of accountability.

An important example is the failure to press the government and those responsible for the health system to show how effective it was at saving lives and restoring people to health. The question was not whether hospitals were doing what they could – it was how much they were able to help people, even if they did their best. Again, all that was needed was a willingness to ask questions, including the most important one: how many patients admitted to hospitals with Covid-19 had recovered *because of the treatment they received*? This might need specific questions to get at the truth: obvious ones were how many patients recovered after being admitted to intensive care, placed on ventilators or received oxygen in other ways. The questions were never asked, although occasionally they were answered.

On only one occasion was the government held to account for its treatment of a Covid-19 patient. That this happened at all had nothing to do with independent initiative – it was again a reaction to digital media or official announcements or both. Shonisani Lethole, a Gauteng businessman, lost his life to Covid-19 after being admitted to Tembisa Hospital. Before he died, Lethole complained of his treatment on digital media and his case was referred to the Health Ombudsman, Professor Malegapuru Makgoba, who found that the hospital was negligent. Among other breaches, Lethole was not offered food for 100 hours after his admission. The Gauteng health department responded that it would suspend the hospital's chief executive officer.[22]

But, as important as Lethole's case was, the reporting did not address the effectiveness of hospital care in treating Covid-19 because the crucial questions which would have thrown light on this were never asked. What treatment were Covid-19 patients at Tembisa receiving? How many had recovered as a result? Questions of this sort would have enabled readers, listeners and viewers to get a sense of whether the hospital would have been able to save Lethole if it had treated him as it should have. Because they were not asked, the incident was treated as purely an example of government neglect, not a window into how much hospitals could do for Covid-19 patients.

This case appeared, however, to have worried Gauteng enough for it to respond with a public relations effort. At the time the Tembisa revelations were circulating in the media, the provincial government held a media briefing on its response to Covid-19 which included a presentation by Professor Mervyn Mer, principal specialist in critical care and pulmonology at Charlotte Maxeke Johannesburg Academic Hospital. His talk contained no hard information and little if any explanation on how effective hospital care was. Instead, it painted the hospital in self-congratulatory terms which even the most ardent publicist might have found excessive. According to Mer, dealing with Covid-19 had 'advanced critical care in Gauteng by up to 20 years'. The 'fast-tracked' acquisition of ventilators and CPAP (continuous positive airway pressure) machines meant that for years to come, 'patients in this province are going to benefit'. The new devices had 'revolutionised care offered and saved countless lives'. South Africa was among the first in the world to have introduced the use of corticosteroids in the treatment of Covid-19 patients, 'to help improve [their] outcome ... long before the evidence became available based on work done in South Africa'.[23]

Mer's presentation contained numerous references to his and the hospital's care for patients including an account of how a patient who knew he was dying was offered his last wish of seeing a final sunset. But he was not forthcoming on any detail of how many patients had been helped to live and how the hospital could be sure it had made a difference. No reporter asked him to support his claim that many lives had been saved with hard evidence or even to elaborate on it despite the fact that official figures showed that 8 087 people had died of Covid-19 in Gauteng at the time that he spoke.[24] Since the speaker was a professor and doctor, it was assumed that what he said must be beyond question – and that, by implication, Covid-19 patients admitted to Gauteng hospitals had a good chance of emerging alive and well.

This was but one example of a trend which became particularly evident when the 'second wave' of infections began to cause great damage. As the year progressed, it became common for the minister of health and doctors to insist that treatment of Covid-19 patients was becoming more effective by the day. This was usually expressed in the claim, repeated time and again, that 'we are learning more about this illness every day'. Given the 'First World' enthusiasm for chemical solutions, Mkhize was particularly excited by the discovery that dexamethasone, a drug which was in plentiful supply in South Africa, was reducing deaths. In August, he said it had reduced fatalities in intensive care units by 25 per cent.[25] This was a more limited breakthrough than he suggested since it obviously meant that three-quarters of ICU patients were not helped. But this and many other statements claiming that health workers were learning more and more about the disease and how to treat it implied that people admitted to hospital had increasing chances of surviving and recovering.

The cheery assurances did not grow nearly as fast as deaths from the virus. It soon became evident that the 'second wave' was far more deadly than the first. Towards the end of January, the SAMRC's report on excess deaths found that 'the weekly number … is more than double the highest number of excess natural deaths of 6 673 reported during the first wave of the pandemic in July'.[26] Official death figures confirmed this trend: they were also more than double those during the height of the 'first wave'. It needed no training in medical science to work out that claims of great improvements in treatment seemed hollow in the face of a worsening death rate. Why South Africans should derive comfort from the news that the health system was getting better at dealing with the disease and that new technological responses to Covid-19 were ushering in a new era of improved health care when their chances of dying from it had more than doubled was never explained. No journalist, politician or civil society organisation asked why the triumphalism of the health system seemed to make people less safe. When I pointed this out in a newspaper column,[27] it was, like other interventions urging the opening of debate on Covid-19,[28] simply ignored.

Throughout the pandemic, information on the progress of the system was always unsolicited – it was released when the minister or the provinces or the hospitals felt it should be. That was not that often, but when it happened at all, the lack of accountability ensured that whoever divulged the information would do so only when they had news to convey which would paint whatever happened, and their role in it, in the best possible light. Even this could sometimes produce less than flattering information. In early March 2021, Groote Schuur Hospital announced proudly that a patient had become the 150th to recover after being ventilated.[29] Given the store placed on ventilators at the start of the pandemic, 150 recoveries did not seem a particularly high number but no one asked how many patients had been placed on ventilators so that they could learn how successful this therapy was. A debate united behind 'readying the health system' showed no interest in how much the system could do to help people.

A predictable accountability failure was the absence of any pressure on the government to work with people in townships – we would not expect 'First World' South Africa to see the 'Third World' as part of a solution. The issue did surface, although in a manner typical of the South African debate. While the 'First World' ignores the concerns of the 'Third', it is aware of its existence. And, while it does not listen to it or learn from it, it knows also that poverty is a problem. While the occasional voice does insist that the poor 'lift themselves up by their bootstraps', it is hard to ignore the reality that much poverty is a consequence of minority rule and apartheid and so this view remains on the margins. And so, participants in the debate invoke 'the poor' in defence of their positions, even when there is no plausible evidence that what they want will help people who are poor. If people living in poverty are victims of government actions which harm them and are not necessary to serve the interests of the 'First World' – when it fails to build houses or manage schooling in townships, for example – the debate is likely to champion their cause, or appear to do so, because it can then do what it usually does: express suburban concerns about government regulation or mismanagement.

This was very much on display during the pandemic. First, as seen in chapter 3, some lockdown opponents invoked the poor to justify their opposition. Gray insisted, inaccurately, that the rules were worsening malnutrition in Soweto. The DA usually remembered to phrase its opposition to the lockdown by insisting that the poor or 'the most vulnerable' would suffer most.[30] It was common for voices denouncing constraints on business or suburban residents to invoke the interests of 'the poor'. In a similar dynamic, at least some in the 'First World' identified with 'Third World' victims of heavy-handed lockdown enforcement,[31] partly, perhaps, because it undermined the credibility of restrictions they disliked.

But none of this meant that the majority were being recognised as partners in the fight against the virus. Either they were used as convenient props to support an argument or their victimhood reinforced the 'First World' view that it was being told what to do by a government which, in its view, should be doing what it told it to do. Even where anger at violence by soldiers was born of concern, it remained consistent with a view which saw townships and shack settlements as places where events happened to people, not where people may be capable of working with the authorities to protect themselves.

Finally, the widespread acceptance among those capable of holding the government to account that high numbers of cases and deaths were inevitable, ensured that there was no pressure on it to act more decisively against Covid-19 when this seemed to be urgently needed. This was particularly evident during periods of 'low transmission' – the period during which, as the Introduction noted, case numbers were around 1 600 a day.

The South African mainstream's idea of an acceptable level of infection is illustrated by the fact that, during this period, South Korea warned of an impending crisis because it reported around 200 daily cases for several days,[32] while in 2021 New Zealand locked down when two cases were discovered because one patient had contracted a more infectious strain.[33] The debate seemed implicitly to accept that even countries which have kept cases and deaths very low were being engulfed by a 'second wave', despite the fact that their earlier successes meant that they became alarmed when they faced a fraction of South Africa's cases at its point of lowest transmission. And so there was no pressure to test and trace effectively when case numbers were low enough to allow this, which made the further spread of the virus, and mutations which might be harder to contain, inevitable. But, even during periods of high transmission, pressure to test and trace was non-existent.

MISSING THE TARGET

There was one medical issue on which the debate did hold the government to account. Again, this illustrated forcefully that responses to the virus reflected the country's internal divide.

It was noted earlier that, not long after vaccines were approved for use in rich countries, medical scientists, cheered on by the media and other 'First World' institutions, began denouncing the government for not buying vaccines early. Madhi and Dasoo were in the front line.[34] This time Gray was on the other side of the fence because she played a senior role in the initial 'roll out' of vaccines (because approval for the regulator could not be obtained quickly for the Johnson and

Johnson vaccine, the initial distribution was a clinical trial and Gray was the company's co-principal investigator).[35] In essence, the complaint against the government by the scientists and the media was that vaccines were the 'only' way out of the pandemic and that it should have 'taken risks' by buying up millions of doses in advance.[36]

That the voices which insisted that only vaccines could help were also those that denounced the lockdown was not an accident. Vaccines are a product of curative medicine and so they were trusted while public health measures were not. The country which first approved vaccines and began to distribute them was the United Kingdom, seen by many in 'First World' South Africa as the centre of the universe. The DA touted vaccines as an alternative to restricting activity, claiming that there was no need for restrictions if vaccines were administered.[37] Vaccines were a convenient 'quick fix' to ensure that the DA's constituency no longer needed to do what the ANC government told it to do.

Pressure on the government to distribute vaccines was, in principle, appropriate: vaccines are much more likely to help people than abandoning public health measures. The vaccines are safe and they do protect against disease and death. But the claim that they were the only way to respond to the pandemic seemed to say more about a bias towards particular types of medicine than about reality. At the time it was made, it was not yet clear whether the vaccines prevented transmission of the virus and, even if they did, it would be months or even years until enough people were vaccinated across the globe to declare the virus defeated. Public health measures were as necessary as ever even after vaccines were distributed and countries such as Chile faced a severe outbreak of the pandemic even after an effective mass vaccination programme.[38] The denunciation of the government as inept buffoons who were incapable of ordering vaccines, standard fare for the 'First World' debate, became so widely accepted that it was stated as indisputable fact by international news media.[39] But it failed to grasp the irony that the government was late in buying vaccines because the debate made this inevitable.[40]

Wealthy countries bought up large stocks of vaccine before clinical trials revealed that they were safe and effective. Their superior bargaining power, and their ability to put aside large sums of money, enabled them to do this. Since the government's accusers saw these countries as exemplars of excellence, they wanted South Africa to do the same. They did not say this until it was too late but it is not unusual for the government to be denounced for not doing things no one in the debate urged it to do before it was assumed to be too late for effective action. It was being told that, in hindsight, it should have bought up large quantities of vaccine at a time when it was not yet clear that any would be developed. Had the medical breakthrough not been achieved and the government had done what the critics demanded, it would have been roundly denounced for setting aside large amounts of cash for a remedy which did not exist. A constant mantra of some government critics is that it is not committed enough to cutting spending – the vaccine purchase would have been ridiculed as an absurd and costly vanity project.

A prime example of denouncing the government for not doing what it would have been attacked for doing was a column by the former editor of a financial newspaper, headlined, in part, 'Hello, useless ANC'.[41] He reported speaking to an executive at the Moderna pharmaceutical company who said it could supply South Africa 40 million doses by the middle of the year. When he wrote this, the government was being blamed for not making vaccines available immediately. If it had placed the order he recommended, it would have been pilloried for making the country wait five months. Oddly for a financial journalist, he did not say how much the doses cost. The price might have been high enough to trigger another assault on 'wasteful expenditure'.

The government had a further option. It could have used its membership of the BRICS alliance to secure Russian or Chinese vaccines. But neither country had published the results of clinical trials at the time it was meant to have been negotiating with them – the Russians only did this in early 2021. The South African Health Products Regulatory Authority (SAHPRA), the country's regulator for medicines, would not have licensed them for use because it needs to see full reports of clinical trials before allowing any medication to be used. Unless the government bullied SAHPRA into dropping its standards, this option was not available. It can be safely assumed that scientists and politicians would have been insulting it on the evening news if government had bullied SAHPRA. The government would also have been blamed if they did not offer protection, as many Western scientists expected when they were in production (the ineffectiveness of the Chinese vaccine, widely used in Chile, is identified by some analyses as one possible reason why Covid-19 continued to affect it severely after it rolled out vaccines).[42] By March 2021, it was still not clear whether Russian or Chinese vaccines are effective against the variant of the virus circulating in South Africa. If they are not, reaction to the government buying vaccines which did not work would have been loud and angry.

Illustration of these points was provided by an incident mentioned earlier – the government bought 1.5 million doses of the AstraZeneca vaccine despite the fact that scientists had identified a new variant of the virus in South Africa against which it might not be effective. Had it waited to find out about this vaccine's effectiveness, it would have been blamed and so it did not wait. In the event, a clinical trial conducted by a team led by Madhi found it was not effective in preventing mild and moderate disease. The government decided not to use the vaccine. It was promptly denounced by a 'mortified' Madhi who said it may work to curb disease and death.[43] This incident became even more bizarre when Madhi wrote an opinion piece chiding the government for not using the AstraZeneca vaccine despite the fact that the WHO had recommended it (needless to say, he did not chide it for ignoring the WHO advice that 'containment' was the priority, not 'mitigation'). He claimed 'a strong biologically plausible reason to expect the AstraZeneca vaccine will protect against severe disease' among patients infected with the variant found in South Africa.[44]

Two aspects made this intervention odd. First, Madhi wrote that 'local scientists' had found that the virus did not prevent mild and moderate disease. But a month earlier he had been interviewed by BBC Radio 4 as the leader of the study and has been repeatedly identified as the study leader. In that interview, he said, 'there's still some hope that the AstraZeneca vaccine might well perform as well as the Johnson & Johnson vaccine in a different age demographic that are at highest risk of severe disease'.[45] Why Madhi did not mention that he led the study is unclear (besides the obvious possibility that, if you are arguing that a study does not matter, you would not want to be identified as its leader). More important is the difference between the BBC interview on the one hand, and his later newspaper interview and opinion article. The later ones imply that, had the government asked for his opinion, he would have told them that there was a 'strong biologically plausible' reason for using it. But that is not what he said to the BBC – 'there's still some hope' suggests that prospects don't look promising. What might he have said about a government which ignored a disappointing clinical trial and administered a vaccine simply because there was 'still some hope' that it might work?

It is also worth noting, given that scientists and the debate increasingly suggest that 'First World' scientists are being frustrated by a 'Third World' government, that the decision not to use the vaccine was not taken by bureaucrats determined to ignore scientific advice – it was a recommendation by scientists. The government was advised not to administer the vaccine by the MAC on Vaccines, whose chair, Barry Schoub, vigorously defended the decision, arguing that there was no value in using the vaccine because it was not effective against the dominant variant in South Africa.[46] Madhi's dispute was, in reality, not one between him and the government at all, although that is how it was portrayed by the media: it was an argument with his fellow scientists.

The incident confirmed much of the absurdity of the debate. Under pressure to buy vaccines, the government persuaded the Serum Institute of India to sell it the doses. No one, including the scientists, urged it to wait because a variant had been identified which the vaccine might not protect against. Only after it bought them did a scientific trial, accompanied by the usual media fanfare, cast doubts on its efficacy. Had the government decided to use the vaccine and it had proved unable to combat severe disease and death, it would have been buried under an avalanche of rage. And, since 'First World' South Africa is fond of using legal action to fight its battles, it could well have been sued. Weeks later, the scientist who led the trials declared himself 'mortified' that the government (which in this case meant his fellow scientists) had drawn an obvious conclusion from them – and from his own remarks. Madhi's later denunciation was given prominent and uncritical media coverage. No one bothered to ask how 'there is still some hope' became 'strongly plausible' or why it took him almost a month to complain. And only when Schoub issued his defence of the decision did media coverage reflect the fact that the government's decision to not use the vaccine was a response to scientific advice.

In a pattern often repeated in the debate, the only certainty was that the government would be blamed whatever it did because the debate has decided that it is a 'Third World' government. This makes accountability very difficult. It is made even more so by the reality that the debate's participants are wrong about the government – it is as embedded in the 'First World' as they are, which is why it was so eager to appease them. This sets up a deeply counter-productive cycle. The government avoided action to buy vaccines because it did not want to be yelled at by the debate but was yelled at anyway. It then acted to show its 'First World' credentials by heeding scientific advice to withdraw the vaccine, only to be yelled at for 'following the science'. Its discomfort did not, however, last long. The debate's deep lack of interest in fighting Covid-19 soon overcame its enthusiasm for denouncing the government, and pressure on it to secure vaccines and distribute them abated when case numbers declined to pre- 'second wave' levels. While the 'second wave' had hurt the suburbs more than the first, it was forgotten the moment it ended.

At every stage of the process, the 'bumbling and inept' government could credibly insist that it was 'following the science' – the science which says that it makes no sense to buy vaccines which do not yet exist or to buy vaccines whose clinical trials have not been published, or that, once vaccines are available, they should be bought as quickly as possible, or that, if clinical trials are said to show that a vaccine is not effective, it should not be used. The outcome was predictable – a vaccine roll-out programme which, by the beginning of May 2021, had failed to offer a vaccine to anyone who was not a health worker, while a 'third wave' was feared to be only weeks away.

BLAMING THE VICTIM

One group of South Africans were very firmly held accountable for the spread of Covid-19: citizens, particularly those living in poverty.

As early as June, after restrictions were reduced amid rising infections and the country moved to lockdown level 3, Ramaphosa said that 'our prevention response is now largely focused on the simple everyday things that each of us can do to protect ourselves and our communities. It is about each of us taking personal responsibility ... for curbing the spread of the disease.'[47] While the government was later forced, very late in the year, to increase restrictions as the virus spread rapidly, shifting responsibility to citizens remained its approach from the time he made these remarks. It remained deeply ingrained in the messages officialdom sent to citizens, regardless of party affiliation. In

March 2021, in a statement which said that a 'third wave' of infections was inevitable, Western Cape premier Winde said: '... it is imperative that we all take personal responsibility to ensure that we remain safe'. His statement's headline described personal responsibility as the 'key' to the fight against the virus.[48] Instead of using a time when cases were low to make test and trace work, it was used to blame the victims and shift responsibility for fighting the virus to them.

The scientists joined in the chorus. Asked in late 2020 whether a 'second wave' was imminent, Karim said that 'how citizens behave will be the ultimate marker for what happens next'. He and Gray, who now publicly adopted the same position despite the earlier media suggestions that they were polar opposites, warned that the virus would spread if 'people become complacent while on holiday and they stop wearing their masks and not do social distance' and if 'they start going to parties'. They were also 'worried about intergenerational family gatherings, children are meeting their parents and grandparents and putting the elderly at risk'. Karim declared: 'We have to control our own behaviour if we do not want to be in a second wave in January.'[49] So too did the media and the rest of the public debate. When the Eastern Cape (with the Western Cape's Garden Route) became the epicentre of the 'second wave', the virus's spread was blamed on citizens' behaviour, not on the authorities who had done nothing to stop the spread.[50]

This ended any prospect of any power holder, public or private, being responsible for case numbers and deaths. If the virus spread and claimed lives, it was not the fault of inadequate testing and tracing, or an inability to ensure that businesses observed the rules, or a refusal to impose restrictions where these were needed. It could not be blamed on policies which failed to offer people in poverty the financial and other support they required to avoid harm. And it was certainly not the fault of an approach by the government and the always adored scientists which gave up before the battle started and was firmly focused on Western realities rather than the resources which were available among South Africans. It was the fault of an errant population which refused to do as it was told.

The human cost of this responsibility-shifting was graphically illustrated by a report compiled for the Eastern Cape government by the HSRC and Walter Sisulu University. It was conducted by the anthropologist Leslie Bank, with Mark Paterson and Nelly Vuyokazi Sharpley.[51] Bank and his colleagues noted that the Eastern Cape was not only the region worst hit in the 'second wave' but was also stigmatised as 'ground zero' for the more infectious strain of the virus. This enabled British media and politicians to deflect attention from their country's failure to curb the virus by creating a widespread panic about the 'South African variant', despite the fact that only a few cases were detected in the United Kingdom.

But the colonial prejudices were not restricted to the British. Bank and his colleagues argue that the Eastern Cape (which in the mind of the debate is as firmly associated with the 'Third World' as the Western Cape is with the 'First') had been stigmatised from March 2020, when Mkhize travelled there to reprimand the provincial government for inadequate testing. It was the only province so blamed despite the fact that test and trace failed everywhere. The BBC focused on the poor state of its hospitals. It suffered severely during the 'second wave' – the research team's informants said that they had never recalled so much death, even during the worst ravages of apartheid and the AIDS epidemic. Its experience confirmed every 'First World' prejudice about the incapacity of the 'Third World'. The province's government joined the 'First World' chorus by blaming the citizenry.[52]

Bank and his colleagues show that it was not the people of the Eastern Cape, with their 'Third World' proclivities, who were to blame – it was the government and its distinctly 'First World' prejudices. During the 'first wave', the government 'suggested that rural funerals and customary practices in the Eastern Cape, rather than urban congestion, township taverns and overcrowded taxis' were the problem. There was 'virtual hysteria' in the media about 'the need to shut down funerals and traditional ceremonies (while Christian church services were hardly mentioned)'. This triggered a 'harsh crackdown' across the region, 'as the police swept through the countryside overturning beer drums, shutting down initiation schools and dispersing mourners at funerals'. The government 'victimised the rural poor and cultivated a culture of fear among them. This was achieved through the closure of hospitals and clinics and the mysterious disappearance of large swathes of the provincial bureaucracy from offices requiring "deep cleaning".' Lockdown restrictions also initially blocked 'the usual Easter flood of migrants back to the countryside, bringing information and gifts from the cities and an important source of labour at harvest time'. (Travel between provinces was not allowed at the beginning of the lockdown.) Villagers believed that they had been abandoned and left trapped amid rising infections. People were left without any medicine, 'except for traditional herbs and remedies they collected themselves'. Alienation was heightened by reports of corruption in the provincial government linked to Covid-19 prevention measures.

Against this background, the 'second wave' arrived. The state had 'retreated' from 'the management of rural life'. Before new restrictions in December, responsibility had been shifted to 'communities and families' and so police were no longer closely monitoring funerals, raiding taverns, checking physical distancing in shopping queues or interfering with customary gatherings. Given the way they had been treated, people were inclined 'to embrace an attitude of defiance, with many families now regrouping in the countryside'. The key trigger to rising infections (after the restriction on travel between provinces ended) was 'the arrival of hundreds of thousands of migrants from the cities, many in overcrowded taxis, as well as the hosting of numerous family reunions and social events'. As the virus spread, 'a deep fear of what happened in local clinics and hospitals' kept people at home rather than at health facilities. Doctors were reduced to begging people to visit hospitals.[53]

No one knows whether the 'South African variant' really did emerge in the Eastern Cape (it might not have emerged in South Africa). But the government's insistence on controlling people rather than working with them – or with the traditional healers on whom many people rely – together with the withdrawal of control when it became too burdensome, ensured both that people wanted to 'restore shattered kinship and social networks'[54] and that there was nothing to stop them. The 'second wave', and the variant it produced, was a product not of the 'backwardness' of the Eastern Cape's citizenry, but of 'First World' belief in the incapacity of the 'Third'. It was the elite, not the people, who enabled the 'second wave' and allowed the virus to mutate in a way which caused more harm.

CHAPTER

5

The Path Not Taken

On 5 March 2021, the anniversary of the first case of Covid-19 identified in South Africa, broadcast media marked the occasion with special programming and a series of particularly fawning interviews with Mkhize and Karim.

The tone was that which we might expect at the celebration of a great achievement. Anecdotes drawn from the official response to the virus were exchanged, and there was a distinctly self-congratulatory air about the discussions. No one seemed willing to spoil the party by pointing out that those whose leadership was being feted had presided over a response which, at that stage, had cost anything from the official figure of some 50 000 lives to the excess death count of more than 138 000[1] and at least 1.5 million cases. Nor did anyone think it noteworthy that, according to official figures, even after the 'second wave' had reportedly swept through the rest of the continent, South Africa had recorded, adjusted for population, almost double the number of cases as Morocco, the second worst affected African country, and

33 times as many as Nigeria, the second worst affected sub-Saharan African country – and that its official death toll, again adjusted for population, was three and a half times Morocco's, 93 times as high as Nigeria's.[2] One broadcaster congratulated the scientists for their 'prescience' in predicting that there would be a severe epidemic.

This response seemed to sum up reality throughout the pandemic. 'First World' South Africa, much like Noah in the biblical account, looked out on its devastated surroundings, so graphically described by Bank in the Eastern Cape,[3] and blamed everyone but itself. Its response was not grief or pain – it was a hearty pat on the back for the government, the scientists, and, presumably, themselves. The reference to 'prescience' seemed to say it all. To use an analogy which would no doubt strike a chord with the 'First World', it was as if a company board had hired a chief executive and a team of consultants to address a challenge. The consultants insisted that financial ruin was inevitable, the chief executive agreed and did nothing to prevent it and, as the firm edged ever closer to the brink, the board congratulated both on predicting the disaster which loomed. They continued to insist that they were superior to other companies whose management and consultants had placed preventing ruin ahead of predicting it.

To sum up what the media and its guests were celebrating, we turn again to Bank, whose summation of the disaster which befell the Eastern Cape applies to the rest of the country too:

> … as the state busily copied best biomedical practices from the global north [where infection rates were skyrocketing], it apparently failed to notice how well the preventative measures of many poorer nations were working. In addition, [it] and its doctors did not stop to ask what rural people felt or thought about Covid-19, nor did they try to communicate with them in their local languages about the nature and impacts of the virus. It was simply assumed that, if South Africa were to keep up with the West, this rural prov-

ince and its country folk would be an obstacle to progress and needed to be hammered into shape by the police with the support of traditional leaders.

So, instead of finding a set of engaged preventative strategies in parts of the country where the health system and infrastructure could not cope with the curative model, the state chose to shame and vilify the rural poor and mock them for their supposed incompetence. A startling example of the way the ANC modernists and medics turned on the majority was provided by their refusal to have anything to do with traditional healers, to whom the majority of the rural population turn for everyday preventative medicines and remedies.[4]

But, while it would surely have been more appropriate to mark the occasion solemnly, as some other countries did, were the media, the government and the scientists not right to assume, as they obviously did, that the illness and death were inevitable? Could South Africa really have been expected to respond like South Korea or New Zealand?

ANOTHER WAY OF SEEING – AND DOING

In one sense, the answer is clearly 'No', the severe epidemic was not inevitable, and 'Yes' the country could have emulated those which kept damage to people to a minimum.

This book has stressed South Africa's experience in relation to the rest of Africa precisely to avoid the objection that what is available to fairly affluent societies in East Asia or Oceania is not available to this country. No one has even attempted a credible explanation of why South Africa did so much more poorly than the rest of the continent. The question has either been ignored or swept under the carpet by BBC-like insistence that the 'dark continent' cannot possibly be better able to deal with an epidemic than some 'First World' countries and that the evidence that it is can be explained away by perpetually hinting at a huge mountain of hidden death and illness which always lacks hard evidence. It is surely not Utopian or fanciful to insist that, with the resources available to it, the country could have done at least as well as others on the continent. A lack of testing and record-keeping might explain an official death toll three or four times that of the next worst affected country. But one 93 times higher?

What South Africa could have done to prevent what happened has been suggested repeatedly in the discussion thus far. For a start, it could have emulated the health minister of Kerala. Having read that a new virus was stalking China, she called her most senior civil servant and asked if the virus would spread to the state. When he said that it would, she immediately called a meeting of senior officials to devise a strategy.[5] While South Africa also called meetings to discuss what to do (although probably not nearly as quickly), the difference was that the purpose of the Kerala meeting was to keep cases and deaths to a minimum, not simply to 'ready the health system' and prepare for many bereavements. Those responsible for public health in the African countries which have kept case and death numbers low surely saw priorities in much the same way.

Covid-19 has challenged the reigning view of what a 'civilised' or 'advanced' society is. Like South Africa's 'First World', the mainstream assumes that these properties describe the rich, more orderly and technologically endowed countries of the global North. But who is more 'civilised' and 'advanced'? The health minister in an Indian state who automatically assumes that her job is to save lives and prevent illness, or the American and Western European governments that were engulfed by the virus because they assumed their first priority was to keep the economy open and inconvenience their citizenry as little as possible? Are South Korea, Taiwan and some states in Africa not more 'advanced' and 'civilised' because they gave greater priority to human life and health? South Africa's response could have been as 'advanced' and 'civilised' as theirs. Its elite, in its desire to show how 'civilised' it was, chose the less civilised path.

This does not mean that fighting Covid-19 is purely an act of will – life does not imitate motivational speakers. But it is surely self-evident that a plan which assumes that many people will fall ill and die whatever is done will ensure that many people fall ill and die. This is not prescience; it is defeatism. At first glance, this seems odd. One of the most persistent themes in the outlook of 'First World' South Africa is a fervent desire to become 'world class'.[6] Huge effort was devoted to ensuring that South African cities achieve this status and its biggest, Johannesburg, describes itself as a 'World Class African City' (the 'African' was only added later on the advice of a British-born municipal official). This obsession covers most aspects of human endeavour and one of its manifestations is a desire to host international conferences and sporting events. At times, it has succeeded despite dire predictions both that its bid would fail and that, when it did not, the event would be catastrophic – two obvious examples are the 2010 football World Cup and the COP17 climate change conference. On the surface, no such ambition to become 'world class' marked its fight against Covid-19. But in reality, this conceit was precisely why the country fared so badly compared to the rest of the continent – its elite was so busy trying to be 'world class' in the curative medicine valued by the West that it produced a response which was substandard for Africa. And it was precisely because 'world class' was code for 'like the rich West countries' that it gave up at the start, for at the core of the desire to be 'world class' lies a deep inferiority complex which assumes that the country will always need to prove itself. Had the elite, including the scientists, had more faith in the capacity of the society in which they live, they might have emulated poorer countries by trying to fight the virus rather than holding it at bay.

Having decided to fight the virus, it might have consulted countries and territories which were showing early successes in keeping cases and deaths low. Obviously, not every idea which works in Korea or Taiwan will work in South Africa. But yet another fixation of the South African elite is the search for models in other parts of the world. People concerned with governance are forever intrigued by German, Canadian or Australian examples of success. While the exemplars are, usually predictably, drawn from 'the West', the economies of the East Asian 'tigers' are often touted as examples to emulate,[7] a continuing theme since the early 1990s. But no similar desire to learn from ways of fighting Covid-19 elsewhere seemed to be evident. The government did insist that it was learning from the WHO, which sent a team to South Africa to assist.[8] But, since its advice on moving from 'containment' to 'mitigation' was largely ignored, the WHO does not seem to have wielded much influence in South Africa. The delegation only visited in August, when the first peak of cases was over.

South Africa's elite could also have sought advice from other African countries. Bernault is not the only source to insist that African experience in dealing with earlier epidemics has imparted public health knowledge which might have eluded both the British media and South African decision-makers but has contributed to ensuring that Covid-19 has done less damage than in South Africa.[9] Yet, as chapter 2 pointed out, no one in a position of responsibility or influence in South Africa seemed to recognise that the rest of the continent may have lessons to teach it.

More specifically, it is trite to point out that lockdowns impose pain and cannot be sustained for long periods. But they do reduce case numbers and deaths. More importantly, they are not needed only or even mainly to ready the health system (whatever that means – no one ever tried to explain how we would recognise a system which was ready). If anything, the South African experience shows that, once the country locked down early, the inevitable result of using lockdowns in this way is to lift restrictions amid rising infections and so ensure that the health system is not ready for anyone – the well-resourced private health system was forced to send patients to public hospitals during the 'second wave'[10] – and to invite mutations which make vaccines less effective. The only way to prevent Covid-19 overwhelming hospitals and mutating is to stop it spreading. Countries which did this locked down early and retained restrictions until the risks of removing them were much lower. While South Africa's retreat from restrictions was portrayed as acceptance of the inevitable, we have seen that it was largely a surrender to lobbies.

We have also seen that there is a way that South Africa could have avoided both an extended lockdown and rising case and death numbers – it could have initiated a test and trace programme which did not rely heavily on an overstretched national laboratory. This, too, has been a key element in the arsenal of countries which have kept case numbers and deaths low. Its failure in South Africa made much of what has been described here unavoidable. The supposedly inevitable choice between 'lives' and livelihoods' was manufactured, not only by the groupthink of the public debate, but by the failure to trace contacts of infected people and to isolate them, which would have made it possible to protect both.

One response to which I have referred only in passing was noticeably absent: an attempt to make it worth people's while to isolate. Experience elsewhere has underlined a trite point: if isolating forces people to lose their incomes, they are unlikely to isolate.[11] The virus is much more likely to be slowed dramatically if people who test positive or who have been in contact with someone who is infected are supported financially if they cannot afford to isolate. South Africa never considered this, presumably because it was thought to be too costly. But, when vaccines became available, R10 billion was set aside to procure them and the contingency reserve was increased by R7 billion to cater for vaccine purchases 'and other emergencies'.[12] In a health emergency, funds can be found. Isolating infected people clearly was a necessary response to a health emergency.

But by far the most important path not taken was that mentioned by Bank and his colleagues' Eastern Cape study – failing to seek a partnership with the citizenry to fight the virus. Throughout the country, South Africa's 'Third World' was treated as a problem to be controlled, not a partner to be enlisted in the fight against Covid-19. An alternative approach would have sought out grassroots organisations and people of influence who could have worked with the government – the traditional healers mentioned earlier are an obvious example. But so are school principals, local clergy and savings club members, who could have been approached and invited to work with the authorities to trace contacts of infected people and help in many other ways. The failure to do this, with the poverty in which many live, ensured that people who wanted to protect themselves often could not. A partnership would have shown sensitivity to those crucial communal ties which, according to the study, were ripped asunder in the Eastern Cape.

To the extent that the South African elite responds to this point, it is to insist, predictably, that the townships lack the capacity to work with authorities to fight the virus. But a tale from the country's not so distant past suggests that surprising reservoirs of capacity can be found if necessary. In 1999, Zola Skweyiya, a constitutional lawyer, was appointed minister of social development.[13] While social grants were formally available to millions of people, only a fraction actually received them. Skweyiya committed his department to ensuring that everyone who was eligible received one. He and his senior officials knew that they had no hope of tracing people on their own and so they turned to churches, schools and local associations and asked them to identify anyone who was entitled to a grant but did not have one. The result was a huge growth in the number of people receiving grants: over the next decade, the number of recipients rose from around 3 million to 13 million – in 2019/20, 18 million people received grants.[14]

An obvious objection is that it is much easier to trace people who will receive a monthly payment than those who will have to isolate to halt the spread of a disease. But we have seen evidence that people in townships and shack settlements were aware that the virus was deadly and wanted to protect themselves from it. They might well have concluded that protection from a deadly virus was a bigger benefit than a grant, particularly if they were paid for doing what they needed to do. There are no doubt other examples of ways in which local people and organisations could have contributed to the fight against Covid-19. Once people are invited to become active participants, remarkable creativity is often unleashed. It is hard to imagine that the fight against Covid-19 would not have been much more effective if grassroots energies and talents had been recruited in its service.

Twice during the course of the pandemic – after the 'first wave' and after the 'second' – South Africa was presented with a chance to end the pain, or at least to reduce its damage. While infection levels remained high by the standards of countries which 'smashed' the curve, they were low enough to allow for an effective test and tracing programme. And both times, by imposing restrictions before case numbers began to rise sharply, the authorities could have prevented illness and death. While the anti-restriction lobby would no doubt complain, the refusal to act ensured that controls on activity would be needed anyway – but that they would come only after illnesses and deaths had begun to rise, leaving the country with the worst of both worlds.

These examples should show that there was an alternative path South Africa could have taken which would have offered a strong chance of reducing deaths and cases. The failure of the national debate to press the government to take any action is surely the lowest point in South Africa's democratic history. While it is often claimed that corruption during the presidency of Jacob Zuma was a democratic failure, the reverse is true:[15] Zuma was defeated by democracy. He and his allies lost power because media exposed them, courts found against them and voters began to desert the governing party. But democracy did not protect the victims of Covid-19 because it did not hold to account anyone with the power to reduce case numbers and deaths. The pandemic spread because of an abject failure of accountability which marks democracy's darkest hour in the past quarter century.

THE BURDEN OF SOCIETY

In another sense, the flood of cases and deaths was inevitable, but not for any of the reasons which the government and the scientists offered.

South Africa was constrained not by the irresistible power of the virus, or its failure to 'follow the science'. The obstacle was, rather, the nature of the society and its division into two worlds, one focused firmly on the West as it looked down on everyone else, the other forced to make do in crowded dwellings and taxis, often deprived of the means to sustain itself, let alone to protect itself.

The defeatism of the government and the scientists and the debate's failure to hold them to account happened not because the government was unaware of the latest public health techniques, or because the scientists read the wrong research papers or because the media and the other voices which shaped the public debate were too stretched to read up on epidemiology and too much in awe of those who had studied it. Their responses were all, in different ways, reflections of the central argument of the book – that South Africa's division into two worlds has survived the end of apartheid and created the multiple failures which shaped the country's response to the pandemic.

While the government and the scientists never said this, their 'defeatism' was born of the deep distrust of the majority of South Africans which tends to characterise the way the 'First World' sees the 'Third'. A workable test and trace programme would have required those who ran it to immerse themselves in the 'Third World' rather than to try to beat it into shape and leave it to its own devices when the beating seemed not to work. The distrust also lay at the heart of the scientists' curious lack of interest in a concerted campaign to reduce cases and deaths.

The debate never seemed to quite understand that fighting Covid-19 was about saving as many lives as possible and keeping as many as well as possible because, after three weeks of lockdown, it did what it always does – it focused on the concerns of the insiders who were not nearly as severely affected as the outsiders and so the return to 'normal' was more important than health and life. For a while, when the 'second wave' began to affect the suburbs, the debate showed some concern but the threat was never great enough to convince it to press the government to fight Covid-19 more effectively. As ever, if the issue was not a huge problem for the insiders, it was no problem at all.

Nor was the fixation with Western Europe and the United States avoidable since this has been a core South African reality for at least a century. The problem was not that the country momentarily forgot that it was in Africa and a part of the global South – the section of society which shapes politics, policy and the public debate has never acknowledged this (in reality, not in the rhetoric some use), so it was hardly likely that it would do this when Covid-19 arrived. This, too, was a product of the divide between the two worlds. We don't know the degree to which 'Third World' South Africa shares the fixation with 'the West' which pervades the 'First'. Since it is associated with wealth and competence, it is possible that most people in townships and shack settlements would gladly share the insiders' preoccupation if poverty and inequality did not deny this to them. But we do know that 'First World' South Africa is focused on the West. This may well have made the response described here inevitable.

South Africa failed to launch a response to Covid-19 which would have maintained cases and deaths at the level experienced by the rest of the continent because the nature of its society, and the politics which this produced, left it far less equipped to deal with the pandemic than countries with far less resources but without the divisions which distracted the gaze of those who take or influence decisions. We don't know precisely why the virus spread far less rapidly and, during 2020, did far less harm to the rest of Africa than expected. But we do know why it did so much more damage in South Africa.

The region which South Africa most closely resembles is not the rest of Africa but Latin America and for much the same reasons. Latin America's high death rates are, according to an editorial in the medical journal *The Lancet*, a consequence of 'longstanding and pervasive inequality – in income, health care, and education – which has been woven into the social and economic fabric of the region'.[16] And in Latin America, too, those who shape the debate look north amidst a southern reality. The Argentine political scientist Guillermo O'Donnell, writing about Latin American intellectuals' expectation under authoritarian rule, observed that their desired democracy was 'the sort ... found in admired countries of the Northwest – admired for their long-enduring regimes and for their wealth, and because both things seemed to go together ... the Northwest was seen as the endpoint of a trajectory ...'.[17] He might have been writing about much of the South African debate. It is no accident that, in both cases, the assumption that the 'Northwest' was 'the endpoint of a trajectory' ensured the response so graphically described by Bank and his colleagues which was, no doubt, mirrored in much of Latin America at the time.

More generally, it is inaccurate to insist that 'First World' countries with their preoccupation with curative medicine all fell victim to high case and death rates. Australia and New Zealand, South Korea and Taiwan do not, for differing reasons, fit the stereotype of 'Third World' countries. But it is surely true that Covid-19 has demonstrated that the notion of an always competent 'First World' and an always needy and incompetent 'Third' is a caricature. In some important areas of life, of which fighting pandemics is one, the skills and tools of the 'First World' lag behind those of the 'Third'. The 'First World' became, as the response of British journalists at the BBC and other news outlets shows, deeply threatened by this prospect. Much of this may be forgotten: once vaccines were discovered, curative medicine and the wealth and power which create it took over, probably ensuring that the countries with the most wealth and influence would be first to protect their populations. But it should not be forgotten. The next pandemic may not be ended by a vaccine and, if it isn't, the public health skills which enabled some countries to avoid huge harm to their citizens will be vital.

South Africa's debate was, arguably, not at all threatened by the prospect that those it dismissed or ignored were better able to protect life and health than 'First World' South Africa. Its belief that it and its concerns are the only ones which matter is so ingrained that reports of 'Third World' competence across the globe were simply brushed off. Since very few voices were interested in highlighting this reality it was sure to be ignored, given the nature of the country's divide and who decides what is important and what is not. There was no attempt in South Africa to show that the rest of Africa was less able to deal with Covid-19: it was simply assumed, despite the evidence to the contrary.

That sums up the nature of South Africa's divisions – and its response to Covid-19. No one wanted many people, particularly in townships and shack settlements, to fall ill and die. No one pressed for the opening of a business or a worship service or an entertainment venue because they did not care that what they wanted to do would destroy the worlds of others. They acted as they did because, in a society with South Africa's divisions, the majority of citizens are as invisible to those whose decisions matter as the continent on which 'First World' South Africa lives. A path which would have vastly reduced the spread of illness and would have saved both lives and livelihoods was possible in theory. In a society still divided, more than a quarter of a century after the formal end of minority rule, between those who can see only the USA and Western Europe, and those who must live with the consequences of their invisibility, what happened was, tragically, bound to happen.

This realisation is crucial not only to how we see fighting Covid-19. The realities which prevented South Africa from keeping it at bay are also those which prevent it from finding a sustainable way to address its economic, social and political challenges. If South Africa is to begin building a society which allows all who live in it to reach their potential, the realities which rendered it unable to protect many people from the virus will need to change. If they do, the country's response to Covid-19 will be seen not as a triumph but as evidence of a burden it so desperately needs to escape.

NOTES

PREFACE

1. Azarrah Karrim and Sarah Evans, 'Unscientific and Nonsensical: Top Scientist Slams Government's Lockdown Strategy', *News24*, 16 May 2020, https://www.news24.com/news24/SouthAfrica/News/unscientific-and-nonsensical-top-scientific-adviser-slams-governments-lockdown-strategy-20200516.
2. Jerome Amir Singh, 'How South Africa's Ministerial Advisory Committee on Covid-19 Can be Optimised', *South African Medical Journal* 110, no. 6 (May 2020): 439–442.
3. Staff Reporter, 'Health Minister Names New Ministerial Advisory Committee on Social Change', *Independent Online*, 17 June 2020, www.iol.co.za/news/politics/health-minister-names-new-advisory-committee-on-social-change-4943171.

INTRODUCTION

1. According to 'Countries in the World by Population (2021)', https://www.worldometers.info/world-population/population-by-country/.
2. Arundhati Roy, 'We Are Witnessing a Crime against Humanity: Arundhati Roy on India's Covid Catastrophe', *The Guardian*, 29 April 2021, https://www.theguardian.com/news/2021/apr/28/crime-against-humanity-arundhati-roy-india-covid-catastrophe.
3. Salim Abdool Karim, 'SA's Covid-19 Epidemic: Trends and Next Steps – Prepared for Minister of Health Zweli Mkhize', Presentation, 13 April 2020; Mia Lindeque, 'SA Can Learn from Europe's Covid-19 Second Wave, Say Experts', *Eyewitness News*, 3 November 2020, https://ewn.co.za/2020/11/03/sa-can-learn-from-europe-s-covid-19-second-wave-say-experts.
4. Zimasa Matiwane and Paige Muller, 'SA Will Have a Severe Epidemic: Prof Salim Abdool Karim', *Business Live*, 23 April 2020, https://www.businesslive.co.za/bd/national/health/2020-04-23-listen-sa-will-have-a-severe-epidemic-prof-salim-abdool-karim/.

5. Department of Health, 'Covid-19 Online Resource and News Portal', https://sacoronavirus.co.za.
6. World Health Organization (WHO), 'WHO Coronavirus Disease (Covid-19) Dashboard', https://covid19.who.int/?gclid=EAIaIQobChMIzJKZ4tGs7QIVjtPtCh04mA8iEAAYASAAEgIVW_D_BwE.
7. Maria Cohut, 'Ill, Abandoned, Unable to Access Help: Living with Long COVID', *Medical News Today*, 7 September 2020, https://www.medicalnewstoday.com/articles/ill-abandoned-unable-to-access-help-living-with-long-covid.
8. Eyewitness News, 'SA Now Has Fifth-Highest Number of Covid-19 Cases in the World', 20 July 2020, https://ewn.co.za/2020/07/20/sa-now-has-fifth-highest-number-of-covid-19-cases-in-the-world.
9. Worldometer, 'Countries Where Covid-19 Has Spread', 3 December 2020, https://www.worldometers.info/coronavirus/countries-where-coronavirus-has-spread/.
10. Calculated from Worldometer, 'Countries Where Covid-19 Has Spread'.
11. See, for example, Al Jazeera, 'Coronavirus Cases in Africa Cross Two Million Mark: AU Tally', 19 November 2020, https://www.aljazeera.com/news/2020/11/19/coronavirus-cases-in-africa-surpass-2-million-reuters-tally.
12. WHO, 'Coronavirus Disease (Covid-19) Dashboard'.
13. Dr Zwelini Mkhize, 'Slideshow: South Africa Covid-19 Experiences to Date', WHO Regional Committee for Africa Meeting: Covid-19 Session, 25 August 2020, https://sacoronavirus.co.za/2020/08/25/slideshow-south-africa-covid-19-experiences-to-date-25th-august-2020/.
14. Calculated using Ineng, 'List of SADC Countries by Population', https://ineng.co.za/list-of-sadc-countries-by-population/.
15. Mkhize, 'Slideshow'.
16. Sylvia Kiwuwa Muyingo, 'Covid-19 Affects Men and Women Differently. It's Important to Track the Data', *Sowetan*, 6 March 2021, https://www.sowetanlive.co.za/news/south-africa/2021-03-06-covid-19-affects-men-and-women-differently-its-important-to-track-the-data/.
17. Alexandra Parker, Gillian Maree, Graeme Gotz and Samkelisiwe Khanyile, *Women and Covid-19 in Gauteng*, August 2020 Map of the Month, Gauteng City-Region Observatory, 1 September 2020.
18. Alexandra Parker, Gillian Maree, Graeme Gotz and Samkelisiwe Khanyile, 'How Covid-19 Puts Women at More Risk than Men in Gauteng, South Africa', *The Conversation*, 21 December 2020, https://theconversation.com/how-covid-19-puts-women-at-more-risk-than-men-in-gauteng-south-africa-150570.
19. Worldometer, 'Coronavirus Egypt', https://www.worldometers.info/coronavirus/country/egypt/.
20. Worldometer, 'Coronavirus', https://www.worldometers.info/coronavirus.
21. Worldometer, 'Coronavirus Nigeria', https://www.worldometers.info/coronavirus/country/nigeria/#:~:text=Nigeria%20Coronavirus%3A%2067%2C557%20Cases%20and%201%2C173%20Deaths%20%2D%20Worldometer.
22. Worldometer, 'Coronavirus'.

Notes

23 Medical Xpress, 'Africa Reports "Hopeful" Daily Drop in Coronavirus Cases', 20 August 2020, https://medicalxpress.com/news/2020-08-africa-daily-coronavirus-cases.html.
24 Max Price, 'Why Don't We Know How Many People Have Been Infected with Covid-19 in South Africa?' *Daily Maverick*, 5 May 2020, https://www.dailymaverick.co.za/article/2020-05-05-why-dont-we-know-how-many-people-have-been-infected-with-covid-19-in-south-africa/.
25 Andrew Harding, 'Coronavirus in South Africa: Scientists Explore Surprise Theory for Low Death Rate', British Broadcasting Corporation, 2 September 2020, https://www.bbc.com/news/world-africa-53998374.
26 Anne Soy, 'Lack of Covid-19 Testing Undermines Africa's "Success"', British Broadcasting Corporation, 27 May 2020, https://www.bbc.com/news/world-africa-52801190.
27 BBC, 'The Gravedigger's Truth: Hidden Coronavirus Deaths', 26 July 2020, https://www.bbc.com/news/av/world-africa-53521563.
28 Linda Nordling, '"Our Epidemic Could Exceed a Million Cases" – South Africa's Top Coronavirus Adviser', *Nature*, 24 July 2020.
29 John Owen Nwachukwu, 'Bill Gates Wonders Why Number of Covid-19 Cases, Deaths Are Not High in Africa', *Daily Post*, 26 December 2020, https://dailypost.ng/2020/12/26/bill-gates-wonders-why-number-of-covid-19-cases-deaths-are-not-high-in-africa/.
30 Peter Mwai and Christopher Giles, 'Coronavirus: How Fast Is it Spreading in Africa?' BBC, 17 August 2020.
31 Nesrine Malik, 'How Many More Images of Covid Disaster Will it Take to Jolt Rich Countries into Action?' *The Guardian*, 3 May 2021, https://www.theguardian.com/commentisfree/2021/may/03/west-images-covid-disaster-poorer-nations-india-crisisFF.
32 Medical Xpress, 'Africa Reports'.
33 eNCA, 'Mkhize: Coronavirus May Have Infected Nearly 12m South Africans', 16 September 2020, https://www.enca.com/news/mkhize-coronavirus-may-have-infected-nearly-12mn-south-africans.
34 Neil Munshi, Joseph Cotterill and Andres Schipani, 'Coronavirus Second Wave Surges across Africa', *Financial Times*, 17 January 2021, https://www.ft.com/content/3d000093-87a3-48f3-8bb5-4ad9a8316aa1.

CHAPTER 1: One Country, Two Realities

1 Jason Beaubien, 'The Country with the World's Worst Inequality Is …', National Public Radio, 2 April 2018, https://www.npr.org/sections/goatsandsoda/2018/04/02/598864666/the-country-with-the-worlds-worst-inequality-is.
2 Aryn Baker, 'What South Africa Can Teach Us as Worldwide Inequality Grows', *Time*, 2 May 2019, https://time.com/longform/south-africa-unequal-country.
3 Thomas Piketty, *Capital in the Twenty-First Century* (Cambridge, MA: Harvard University Press, 2014).

4   Johns Hopkins University Coronavirus Resource Centre (JHU), 'Covid-19 Dashboard', https://coronavirus.jhu.edu/map.html.
5   See, for example, David Yudelman, *The Emergence of Modern South Africa: State, Capital and the Incorporation of Organized Labor on the South African Gold Fields, 1902–1939* (Cape Town: David Philip, 1984).
6   Richard Turner, 'Black Consciousness and White Liberals', *Reality*, July 1972, p.20.
7   Hermann Giliomee, 'An Extraordinary Country', in *The Last Afrikaner Leaders: A Supreme Test of Power* (Charlottesville: University of Virginia Press, 2012), 17–37.
8   Cited in T. Dunbar Moodie, *The Rise of Afrikanerdom: Power, Apartheid and Afrikaner Civil Religion* (Berkeley: University of California Press, 1980), 266.
9   Steven Friedman, *Prisoners of the Past: South African Democracy and the Legacy of Minority Rule* (Johannesburg: Wits University Press, 2021).
10 Steven Friedman, 'Seeing Ourselves as Others See Us: Racism, Technique and the Mbeki Administration', in *Mbeki and After: Reflections on the Legacy of Thabo Mbeki*, ed. Daryl Glaser (Johannesburg: Wits University Press, 2010), 163–186.
11 Haroon Bhorat, Aalia Cassim and Alan Hirsch, *Policy Co-Ordination and Growth Traps in a Middle-Income Country Setting: The Case of South Africa*, WIDER Working Paper 2014/155 (Helsinki: United Nations University World Institute for Development Economics Research, 2014).
12 James Moulder, 'The Predominantly White Universities: Some Ideas for a Debate', in *Knowledge and Power in South Africa*, ed. Jonathan Jansen (Johannesburg: Skotaville, 1991), 117, 118.
13 Anye Nymanjoh, 'The Phenomenology of *Rhodes Must Fall*: Student Activism and the Experience of Alienation at the University of Cape Town', *Strategic Review for Southern Africa* 39, no. 1 (May 2017): 256–277.
14 Statistics South Africa, 'Mid-Year Population Estimates 2019', *Statistical Release* P0302, 29 July 2019.
15 Statistics South Africa, *Key findings: P0277 – Quarterly Employment Statistics (QES)*, September 2020.
16 The term 'immediate dependents' here means nuclear family members – spouses, children and grandchildren. It is important to emphasise this because many black working people are expected to contribute to the incomes of unemployed extended family members and others who depend on them for a portion of their income. These dependents are outsiders since they depend on the generosity of wage and salary earners. Immediate dependents are insiders because their claim on a portion of the income is grounded in law.
17 Aubrey Matshiqi, 'Why Manuel Is Right and Wrong about Manyi's "Racism"', *Business Day*, 8 March 2011, http://www.businessday.co.za/articles/Content.aspx?id=136509.
18 Richard Humphries, Thabo Rapoo and Steven Friedman, 'The Shape of the Country: Negotiating Regional Government', in *The Small Miracle: South Africa's Negotiated Settlement*, eds Steven Friedman and Doreen Atkinson (Johannesburg: Ravan Press, 1994), 148–181.

19 Deborah Brautigam, 'Contingent Consent: Export Taxation and State Building in Mauritius', Paper presented at the annual meeting of the American Political Science Association, Marriott, Loews Philadelphia, and the Pennsylvania Convention Center, Philadelphia, PA, 31 August 2006.
20 African National Congress, 'MYANC: More Jobs, More Decent Jobs', *2019 Election Manifesto*, https://www.anc1912.org.za/myanc-more-jobs-more-decent-jobs-httpstcoj1hes0kftg.
21 Allan Greenblo, 'Social Grant System Has Failed to Uplift South Africans', *Business Day*, 15 July 2019, https://www.businesslive.co.za/fm/opinion/2019-07-15-allan-greenblo-social-grant-system-has-failed-to-uplift-south-africans/; Africa Check, 'Factsheet: Social Grants in South Africa', 28 February 2017, https://africacheck.org/fact-checks/factsheets/factsheet-social-grants-south-africa-separating-myth-reality.
22 Mandla Seleoane, 'Resource Flows in Poor Communities: A Reflection on Four Case Studies', in *Giving & Solidarity: Resource Flows for Poverty Alleviation in South Africa*, eds Adam Habib and Brij Maharaj (Cape Town: HSRC Press, 2008), 121–158.
23 Leila Patel, Yolanda Sadie, Victoria Graham, Aislinn Delaney and Kim Baldry, *Voting Behaviour and the Influence of Social Protection: A Study of Voting Behaviour in Three Poor Areas of South Africa* (Johannesburg: Centre for Social Development in Africa and Department of Politics, University of Johannesburg, June 2014).
24 Estelle Ellis, 'Gender-Based Violence Is South Africa's Second Pandemic, Says Ramaphosa', *Daily Maverick*, 18 June 2020, https://www.dailymaverick.co.za/article/2020-06-18-gender-based-violence-is-south-africas-second-pandemic-says-ramaphosa/.
25 Sihle Mlambo, 'SA Nominates Cuban Doctors for Nobel Peace Prize, DA and Action SA Not Pleased', *Independent Online*, 2 February 2021, https://www.iol.co.za/news/south-africa/gauteng/sa-nominates-cuban-doctors-for-nobel-peace-prize-da-and-action-sa-not-pleased-ca3c8870-1eae-4f89-aa3a-35a9d047d522.
26 Karl von Holdt, 'South Africa: The Transition to Violent Democracy', *Review of African Political Economy* 40, no. 138 (2013): 589–604.

CHAPTER 2: Following the Science

1 Philip Machanik, 'Covid-19: Free the Evidence', *Mail and Guardian*, 9 July 2020, https://mg.co.za/coronavirus-essentials/2020-06-09-covid-19-free-the-evidence/.
2 Peter Hotez, 'Anti-Science Kills: From Soviet Embrace of Pseudoscience to Accelerated Attacks on US Biomedicine', *PLoS Biol* 19, no. 1 (2021): e3001068, https://doi.org/10.1371/journal.pbio.3001068.
3 Jason Weismueller, Jacob Shapiro, Jan Oledan and Paul Harrigan, 'Coronavirus Misinformation Is a Global Issue, but which Myth You Fall for Likely Depends on Where You Live', *The Conversation*, 11 August 2020, https://theconversation.

4. William Wallis and Jasmine Cameron-Chileshe, 'UK Community Leaders Battle Vaccine Scepticism among Ethnic Minorities', *Financial Times*, 1 February 2021, https://www.ft.com/content/9019eddf-6d65-4b8d-b7b3-241578dc6e4f.
5. Business Tech, 'South Africa's State of Disaster Extended by Another Month', 14 April 2021, https://businesstech.co.za/news/trending/483119/south-africas-state-of-disaster-extended-by-another-month-2/.
6. Refilwe Pitjeng, 'Covid-19: What Exactly Is the National Command Council?' *Eyewitness News*, 4 May 2020.
7. SA News, 'New Committee to Focus on Covid-19 Vaccine for South Africa', *BusinessTech*, 15 September 2020, https://businesstech.co.za/news/trending/433571/new-committee-to-focus-on-covid-19-vaccine-for-south-africa/.
8. Marcus Low and Nathan Geffen, 'Here's What the Models Predict about Covid-19', *GroundUp*, 22 May 2020, https://www.groundup.org.za/articles/heres-what-models-predict-about-covid19.
9. South African Government, 'Covid-19 Models', https://www.gov.za/covid-19/models/covid-19-models#.
10. Steven Friedman, 'Gaining Comprehensive Aids Treatment in South Africa: The Extraordinary "Ordinary"', in *Citizen Action and National Policy Reform*, eds John Gaventa and Rosemary McGee (London: Zed Books, 2010), 44–68.
11. Nathan Geffen, *Echoes of Lysenko: State-Sponsored Pseudo-Science in South Africa*, CSSR Working Paper No. 149 (Cape Town, Centre for Social Science Research, Aids and Society Research Unit, March 2006).
12. Carien du Plessis, 'How South Africa's Action on Covid-19 Contrasts Sharply with its Response to Aids', *The Guardian*, 27 March 2020, https://www.theguardian.com/global-development/2020/may/27/how-south-africas-action-on-covid-19-contrasts-sharply-with-its-response-to-aids-coronavirus.
13. Cyril Ramaphosa, 'South Africa's Risk Adjusted Strategy to Manage Spread of Coronavirus Covid-19', South African Government, 15 August 2020, https://www.gov.za/speeches/president-cyril- August 15 2020.
14. Kevin Brandt, 'Ramaphosa: Covid-19 Screening Drive Will be Intensive and Far-Reaching', *Eyewitness News*, 31 March 2020, https://ewn.co.za/2020/03/31/ramaphosa-covid-19-screening-drive-will-be-intensive-and-far-reaching.
15. Mandisa Mbali, 'Mbeki's Denialism and the Ghosts of Apartheid and Colonialism for Post-Apartheid AIDS Policy-Making', Workshop Paper presented at University of Natal, Durban, School of Development Studies, 15 April 2002, www.hivan.org.za/admin/documents/Mbeki's20%denialism.doc.
16. Iavan Pijoos, 'How to Protect Yourself from Airborne Transmission of Covid-19', *Times Live*, 9 July 2020, https://www.timeslive.co.za/news/south-africa/2020-07-09-how-to-protect-yourself-from-airborne-transmission-of-covid-19/.
17. The acronym stands for 'susceptible, infected and recovered or removed'.
18. Michael Gering and Mojalefa Ralekhetho, 'Walking through the Pandemic Modelling, Exponential Growth and Herd Immunity Maze', *Daily Maverick*,

8 October 2020, https://www.dailymaverick.co.za/opinionista/2020-10-08-walking-through-the-pandemic-modelling-exponential-growth-and-herd-immunity-maze/.
19　Nina Bai, 'Still Confused about Masks? Here's the Science behind How Face Masks Prevent Coronavirus', UCFS, 26 June 2020, https://www.ucsf.edu/news/2020/06/417906/still-confused-about-masks-heres-science-behind-how-face-masks-prevent.
20　Alexander Winning and Olivia Kumwenda-Mtambo, 'South Africa Puts AstraZeneca Vaccinations on Hold over Variant Data', *Reuters*, 8 February 2021, https://www.reuters.com/article/uk-health-coronavirus-safrica-idUSKBN2A80J2.
21　Jon Cohen, 'South Africa Suspends Use of AstraZeneca's Covid-19 Vaccine after it Fails to Clearly Stop Virus Variant', *Science*, 8 February 2021, https://www.sciencemag.org/news/2021/02/south-africa-suspends-use-astrazenecas-covid-19-vaccine-after-it-fails-clearly-stop.
22　Madeleine Hoecklin, 'Switzerland Nixes AstraZeneca Vaccine until More Evidence Is Obtained. Other EU Countries Rule out Vaccine for Older People', *Health Policy Watch*, 4 February 2021, https://healthpolicy-watch.news/switzerland-nixes-astrazeneca-vaccine-until-more-evidence-is-obtained-other-eu-countries-rule-out-vaccine-for-older-people/.
23　Talha Khan Burki, 'Herd Immunity for Covid-19', *The Lancet Respiratory Medicine* 9, no. 2 (November 2020): 135–136.
24　Joscha Bach, 'Don't "Flatten the Curve," Squash it!' *Medium*, 14 March 2020, https://medium.com/@joschabach/flattening-the-curve-is-a-deadly-delusion-eea324fe9727.
25　Singh, 'Ministerial Advisory Committee', 1.
26　Oupa Lehulere, 'Scientists against Science: The Campaign to Open "the Economy" in the Time of Covid-19', *Karibu*, 5 June 2020, https://karibu.org.za/scientists-against-science-the-campaign-to-open-the-economy-in-the-time-of-covid-19/.
27　Matiwane and Muller, 'SA Will Have a Severe Epidemic'.
28　Karim, 'Trends and Next Steps', Slide 25.
29　Karim, 'Trends and Next Steps', Slide 10, Slide 4.
30　Karim, 'Trends and Next Steps', Slide 18.
31　Katherine Childs, 'SA's Covid-19 Models Were "Flawed", Says Former NICD Expert', *Business Live*, 24 April 2020, https://www.businesslive.co.za/fm/features/2020-04-24-sas-covid-19-models-were-flawed-says-former-nicd-expert/.
32　Beth Amato, 'Second Wave Severity: What Semi-Saved South Africa?' University of the Witwatersrand, Johannesburg, https://www.wits.ac.za/news/latest-news/research-news/2021/2021-01/second-wave-severity-what-semi-saved-south-africa.html.
33　National Institute for Communicable Diseases, 'Latest Confirmed Cases of Covid-19 in South Africa (24 Jan 2021)', https://www.nicd.ac.za/latest-confirmed-cases-of-covid-19-in-south-africa-24-jan-2021/.

34 South African Medical Research Council (SAMRC), 'Report on Weekly Deaths in South Africa', https://www.samrc.ac.za/reports/report-weekly-deaths-south-africa.
35 Karrim and Evans, 'Unscientific and Nonsensical'.
36 Karrim and Evans, 'Unscientific and Nonsensical'.
37 Jeremy Baskin, 'The Coming Covid Science Sh*tstorm: Responding to the Great Barrington Declaration', *Arena Online*, 15 October 2020, https://arena.org.au/the-coming-covid-science-shtstorm-responding-to-the-great-barrington-declaration/.
38 Baskin, 'The Coming Covid Science'.
39 Owen Matthews, 'Britain Drops its Go-it-Alone Approach to Coronavirus', *Foreign Policy*, 17 March 2020, https://foreignpolicy.com/2020/03/17/britain-uk-coronavirus-response-johnson-drops-go-it-alone/.
40 Statista, 'Coronavirus (Covid-19) Deaths Worldwide per One Million Population as of February 4, 2021, by Country', https://www.statista.com/statistics/1104709/coronavirus-deaths-worldwide-per-million-inhabitants/.
41 Statista, 'Cumulative Number of Coronavirus (Covid-19) Cases in the Nordic Countries (as of February 2, 2021)', https://www.statista.com/statistics/1102257/cumulative-coronavirus-cases-in-the-nordics/; 'Cumulative Number of Coronavirus (Covid-19) Deaths in the Nordic Countries (as of February 2, 2021)', https://www.statista.com/statistics/1113834/cumulative-coronavirus-deaths-in-the-nordics/.
42 Sam Bowman, 'Is Rishi Sunak the Most Dangerous Man in Government?' *The Guardian*, 8 February 2021, https://www.theguardian.com/commentisfree/2021/feb/05/rishi-sunak-government-pandemic-chancellor.
43 Christie Aschwanden, 'The False Promise of Herd Immunity for Covid-19', *Nature*, 21 October 2020, https://www.nature.com/articles/d41586-020-02948-4
44 Statista, 'Distribution of Coronavirus (Covid-19) Deaths in South Africa as of November 16, 2020, by Age', https://www.statista.com/statistics/1127280/coronavirus-covid-19-deaths-by-age-distribution-south-africa/.
45 Jennifer K. Logue, Nicholas M. Franko, Denise J. McCulloch et al., 'Sequelae in Adults at 6 Months after Covid-19 Infection', *JAMA Network Open* 4, no. 2 (2021): e210830, doi:10.1001/jamanetworkopen.2021.0830.
46 Aschwanden, 'The False Promise'.
47 Laura Spinney, 'How Elimination versus Suppression became Covid's Cold War', *The Guardian*, 3 March 2021, https://www.theguardian.com/commentisfree/2021/mar/03/covid-19-elimination-versus-suppression.
48 Susan M. Malinowski, 'Eight Ways to Smash, Not Just Flatten, the Coronavirus Curve', *Medium*, 2 April 2020, https://susanmmalinowskimd.medium.com/eight-ways-to-smash-not-just-flatten-the-coronavirus-curve-d7b27167d28f; Rachael Rettner, 'Instead of Just Flattening the COVID-19 Curve, Can We "Crush" it?' *Live Science*, 3 April 2020, https://www.livescience.com/can-covid-19-be-crushed.html; Devi Sridhar, 'Crunching the Coronavirus Curve Is Better than Flattening it, as New Zealand Is Showing', *The Guardian*, 22 April 2020, https://www.theguardian.com/commentisfree/2020/apr/22/flattening-curve-new-zealand-coronavirus.

49 World Health Organization, 'Situation reports on COVID-19 outbreak – Sitrep 07, 15 April 2020', External Situation Report 7, data as reported by 14 April 2020, https://www.afro.who.int/publications/situation-reports-covid-19-outbreak-sitrep-07-15-april-2020.
50 Ashwin Palaniappan, Udit Dave and Brandon Gosine, 'Comparing South Korea and Italy's Healthcare Systems and Initiatives to Combat Covid-19', *Pan American Journal of Public Health* 44 (2020): e53. https://doi.org/10.26633/RPSP.2020.53.
51 Emma Smith, 'These Countries Have Only a Handful of Ventilators' *Devex*, 9 April 2020, https://www.devex.com/news/these-countries-have-only-a-handful-of-ventilators-96970.
52 Tiyese Jeranji, 'Covid-19: How Mechanical Ventilation Has Saved Lives at Groote Schuur Hospital', *Spotlight*, 8 September 2020, https://www.spotlightnsp.co.za/2020/09/08/covid-19-how-mechanical-ventilation-has-saved-lives-at-groote-schuur-hospital.
53 Palaniappan, Dave and Gosine, 'Comparing', 1.
54 World Health Organization Democratic Republic of Congo, 'Building on Ebola Response to Tackle Covid-19 in DRC', 25 June 2020, https://www.afro.who.int/news/building-ebola-response-tackle-covid-19-drc.
55 Florence Bernault, 'Some Lessons from the History of Epidemics in Africa', *African Arguments*, 6 June 2020, https://africanarguments.org/2020/06/some-lessons-from-the-history-of-epidemics-in-africa/.
56 Leslie Bank, 'Ground Zero: Deep-Seated Colonial-Era Prejudice Fuelled the Pandemic in Rural Eastern Cape', *Daily Maverick*, 24 February 2021, https://www.dailymaverick.co.za/article/2021-02-24-ground-zero-deep-seated-colonial-era-prejudice-fuelled-the-pandemic-in-rural-eastern-cape/.
57 Bank, 'Ground Zero'.
58 Anthony Costello, 'Poor Support for Self-Isolation Undermines the UK's Covid Vaccination Effort', *The Guardian*, 10 February 2021, https://www.theguardian.com/commentisfree/2021/feb/10/support-self-isolation-uk-covid-vaccination-effort-virus-replicate-mutations-vaccines. Costello is professor of global health and sustainable development at University College London and a former WHO official.
59 Laura Spinney, 'The Coronavirus Slayer! How Kerala's Rock Star Health Minister Helped Save it from Covid-19', *The Guardian*, 14 May 2020, https://www.theguardian.com/world/2020/may/14/the-coronavirus-slayer-how-keralas-rock-star-health-minister-helped-save-it-from-covid-19.
60 Johns Hopkins University, 'Covid-19 Data Repository by the Center for Systems Science and Engineering (CSSE) at Johns Hopkins University', https://github.com/CSSEGISandData/COVID-19.
61 Indiaonlinepages.com, 'Population of Kerala 2020', http://www.indiaonlinepages.com/population/kerala-population.html.
62 Costello, 'Poor Support'.
63 Tedros Adhanom Ghebreyesus, 'WHO Director-General's Opening Remarks at the Mission Briefing on Covid-19 – 12 March 2020', World Health Organization, 12 March 2020, https://www.who.int/director-general/speeches/

detail/who-director-general-s-opening-remarks-at-the-mission-briefing-on-covid-19—12-march-2020.
64 Nordling, 'Our Epidemic'.
65 Harding, 'Coronavirus in South Africa'.
66 South African Medical Research Council, 'Prof Salim Abdool Karim', https://www.samrc.ac.za/people/prof-salim-abdool-karim.
67 Statistics South Africa, National Household Travel Survey 2013 cited in Ciara Staunton, Carmen Swanepoel and Melodie Labuschaigne, 'Between a Rock and a Hard Place: Covid-19 and South Africa's Response', *Journal of Law and the Biosciences* 7, no. 1 (2020): 1–12, doi:10.1093/jlb/lsaa052.
68 Parker, Maree, Gotz and Khanyile, 'How COVID-19 Puts Women at More Risk'.
69 Kirsten Jacobs, 'Dlamini-Zuma Explains Reasons for Tobacco Ban', *Cape Town etc.*, 27 May 2020, https://www.capetownetc.com/news/dlamini-zuma-explains-reasons-for-tobacco-ban/.
70 Kgomotso Modise, 'Patel Explains Why Cooked Food Can't Be Sold during Lockdown', *Eyewitness News*, 21 April 2020, https://ewn.co.za/2020/04/21/patel-explains-why-hot-food-can-t-be-sold-during-lockdown.
71 Tom Head, 'SA's Alcohol Ban Explained: Why Booze Is Barred during Lockdown', *The South African*, 26 March 2020, https://www.thesouthafrican.com/news/why-alcohol-sale-banned-south-africa-during-lockdown/.
72 Rebecca Davis, 'Unpacking the Rationality of South Africa's Lockdown Regulations', *Daily Maverick*, 14 May 2020, https://www.dailymaverick.co.za/article/2020-05-14-unpacking-the-rationality-of-south-africas-lockdown-regulations/.
73 Luke Daniel, 'Ramaphosa's Decision to Deploy 73 000 Soldiers Questions Lockdown's End', *The South African*, 23 April 2020, https://www.thesouthafrican.com/news/does-ramaphosa-sandf-army-deployment-indicate-a-lockdown-extension/.
74 Iavan Pijoos, '"Beer Poured over His Head, Choked, Kicked, Hit with Machine Gun": How Collin Khosa Died in Alex', *Times Live*, 15 April 2020, https://www.timeslive.co.za/news/south-africa/2020-04-15-beer-poured-over-his-head-choked-kicked-hit-with-machine-gun-how-collin-khosa-died-in-alex/.
75 Emily Mendenhall and Andrew Wooyoung Kim, 'People in Soweto Told Us about Their Fears in the First Weeks of South Africa's Lockdown', *The Conversation*, 8 October 2020, https://theconversation.com/people-in-soweto-told-us-about-their-fears-in-the-first-weeks-of-south-africas-lockdown-142325.
76 Cebelihle Mthethwa, 'South Africa: Coronavirus – Commuters Fear Infection in Overcrowded Taxis, Buses and Trains', *AllAfrica*, 17 March 2020, https://allafrica.com/stories/202003170127.html.
77 Sakhile Ndlazi, 'Covid-19: Back-to-School Fears Mount', *Pretoria News*, 29 April 2020, https://www.iol.co.za/pretoria-news/covid-19-back-to-school-fears-mount-47325768.
78 Karim, 'Trends and Next Steps', Slide 19.

Notes

79   Natasha Berting, 'Innovative Handwashing Stations Pop up across Africa', *What Design Can Do*, 7 May 2020, https://www.whatdesigncando.com/stories/hand-washing-stations-africa/.
80   Setumo Stone, 'Could This Handwashing Station be the Solution to SA's Hygiene Problems?' *City Press*, 1 June 2020, https://www.news24.com/citypress/news/could-this-handwashing-station-be-the-solution-to-sas-hygiene-problems-20200601.
81   The Citizen, 'Medical Experts Slam Govt for Banning Booze but Loading Taxis', 14 July 2020, https://citizen.co.za/news/covid-19/2320867/medical-experts-slam-govt-for-banning-booze-but-loading-taxis/.
82   Marc Mendelson and Shabir Madhi, 'South Africa's Coronavirus Testing Strategy Is Broken and Not Fit for Purpose: It's Time for a Change', *South African Medical Journal* 110, no. 6 (June 2020): 429–431.
83   Marc Mendelson and Shabir Madhi, 'South Africa's Covid-19 Testing Strategy Needs Urgent Fixing: Here's How to Do it', *The Conversation*, 8 May 2020, https://theconversation.com/south-africas-covid-19-testing-strategy-needs-urgent-fixing-heres-how-to-do-it-138225.
84   Mendelson and Madhi, 'Testing Strategy Needs Urgent Fixing'.
85   Mendelson and Madhi, 'South Africa's Coronavirus Testing Strategy', 430.
86   Mendelson and Madhi, 'Testing Strategy Needs Urgent Fixing'.
87   Mendelson and Madhi, 'South Africa's Coronavirus Testing Strategy', 429.
88   Mendelson and Madhi, 'South Africa's Coronavirus Testing Strategy', 429.
89   Shabir A. Madhi, Alex van den Heever, David Francis, Imraan Valodia, Martin Veller and Michael Sachs, 'South Africa Needs to End the Lockdown: Here's a Blueprint for its Replacement', *The Conversation*, 9 April 2020, https://theconversation.com/south-africa-needs-to-end-the-lockdown-heres-a-blueprint-for-its-replacement-136080.
90   Marcia Frellick, 'Fauci: "About 40%–45% of Infections Are Asymptomatic"', *Medscape*, 11 September 2020, https://www.medscape.com/viewarticle/937297.
91   Sangmi Cha and Rocky Swift, 'Symptomless and Spreading, South Korea Battles Surge in Silent Covid-19 Cases', *Reuters*, 27 November 2020, https://www.reuters.com/article/us-health-coronavirus-asymptomatic-asia/symptomless-and-spreading-south-korea-battles-surge-in-silent-covid-19-cases-idUSKBN2870LV.
92   Carl Heneghan, Jon Brassey and Tom Jefferson, 'Covid-19: What Proportion Are Asymptomatic?' The Centre for Evidence-Based Medicine, Oxford University, 6 April 2020, https://www.cebm.net/covid-19/covid-19-what-proportion-are-asymptomatic/.
93   Devi Sridhar, 'As More Local Lockdowns Begin, the Hard Truth Is There's No Return to "Normal"', *The Guardian*, 21 September 2020, https://www.theguardian.com/commentisfree/2020/sep/21/local-lockdowns-begin-no-normal-advice-live-with-covid.
94   Karrim and Evans, 'Unscientific and Nonsensical'.
95   Karrim and Evans, 'Unscientific and Nonsensical'.
96   Spinney, 'Elimination versus Suppression'.
97   Salim Abdool Karim, 'Differences of Opinion Vital "to Arriving at the Best Advice": Prof Abdool Karim', *Sowetan*, 17 May 2020, https://www.sowetanlive.

co.za/news/south-africa/2020-05-17-differences-of-opinion-vital-to-arriving-at-the-best-advice-prof-abdool-karim/.
98 Mia Malan, 'Politicking, Pandemics and Prestige: What's Really behind the Squabbles at South Africa's High-Level Covid-19 Committee?' Bhekisisa Centre for Health Journalism, 19 May 2020, https://bhekisisa.org/article/2020-05-19-ministerial-advisory-committeecommittee-politics-of-science-glenda-gray-salim-abdool-karim-zweli-mkhize.

CHAPTER 3: The Science Unravels

1 South African Government, 'Regulations and Guidelines – Coronavirus Covid-19', 2020, https://www.gov.za/covid-19/resources/regulations-and-guidelines-coronavirus-covid-19?gclid=EAIaIQobChMI1Yr9xZq17wIVEu7tCh0UmQn7EAAYASAAEgIlS_D_BwE#.
2 Juniour Khumalo, 'South Africans Are Now Gatvol of Lockdown', *City Press*, 26 April 2020, https://www.news24.com/citypress/Special-Report/Covid-19_Survey/support-for-lockdown-plummets-20200426.
3 Khumalo, 'South Africans Are Now Gatvol'.
4 Khumalo, 'South Africans Are Now Gatvol'.
5 Tamar Kahn, 'Let More People Go to Work during Lockdown, Institute of Race Relations Urges', *Business Live*, 2 April 2020, https://www.businesslive.co.za/bd/national/health/2020-04-02-let-more-people-go-to-work-during-lockdown-institute-of-race-relations-urges.
6 Africa News Agency (ANA) Reporter, 'Institute of Race Relations Mulls Joining Lockdown Legal Challenges', *Independent Online*, 20 May 2020, https://www.iol.co.za/news/politics/institute-of-race-relations-mulls-joining-lockdown-legal-challenges-48232061.
7 Steven Friedman and Zimitri Erasmus, 'Counting on "Race": What the Surveys Say (and Do Not Say) about "Race" and Redress', in *Racial Redress and Citizenship in South Africa*, eds Adam Habib and Kristina Bentley (Cape Town: HSRC Press, 2008), 33–74.
8 Gareth van Onselen 'We Underestimated How Low Turnout Would Go – IRR', *Politicsweb*, 12 May 2019, https://www.politicsweb.co.za/politics/postelection-poll-analysis—irr.
9 Khumalo, 'South Africans Are Now Gatvol'.
10 Theto Mahlakoana, 'Dlamini Zuma's Reasons for Tobacco Sales Plan Are "All Over the Place", Court Hears', *Eyewitness News*, 10 June 2020, https://ewn.co.za/2020/06/10/dlamini-zuma-s-reasons-for-tobacco-sales-ban-all-over-the-place-court-hears.
11 Emmanuel Tjiya, 'Minister Ebrahim Patel Dictates to Fashion Police', *Sowetan*, 14 May 2020, https://www.sowetanlive.co.za/entertainment/2020-05-14-minister-ebrahim-patel-dictates-to-fashion-police/.
12 Discussions with market analysts, May 2020.
13 Karrim and Evans, 'Unscientific and Nonsensical'.

14 Katharine Child, 'Profile: "It's a Virus, Not War", Says Dr Aslam Dasoo', *Business Live*, 1 October 2020, https://www.businesslive.co.za/fm/fm-fox/2020-10-01-profile-its-a-virus-not-war-says-dr-aslam-dasoo.
15 Karrim and Evans, 'Unscientific and Nonsensical'.
16 News24, 'Zweli Mkhize's Statement on Prof Glenda Gray's Criticism of Lockdown Regulations', 21 May 2020, https://www.news24.com/news24/SouthAfrica/News/read-in-full-zweli-mkhizes-statement-on-prof-glenda-grays-criticism-of-lockdown-regulations-20200521. The fact that Gray's title is mentioned but not Mkhize's could be seen as revealing by people sensitive to racial nuance.
17 Azarrah Karrim, 'I Didn't Criticise the Lockdown, but the Regulations – Prof Glenda Gray after Mkhize Slams Criticism', *News24*, 21 May 2020, https://www.news24.com/news24/SouthAfrica/News/i-did-not-criticise-the-lockdown-but-the-regulations-glenda-gray-after-mkhize-slams-criticism-20200521.
18 Tamar Kahn, 'MRC Board Agrees to Launch Investigation into Glenda Gray', *Business Live*, 25 May 2020, https://www.businesslive.co.za/bd/national/health/2020-05-25-mrc-board-agrees-to-launch-investigation-into-glenda-gray/.
19 Eyewitness News, 'SAMRC Drops Any Further Investigation into Glenda Gray', 26 May 2020, https://ewn.co.za/2020/05/26/samrc-drops-any-further-investigation-into-professor-glenda-gray.
20 Alex Patrick, 'Group of Leading Scientists Come out in Support of Glenda Gray Who Dared to Criticise Lockdown Rules', *Times Live*, 23 May 2020, https://www.timeslive.co.za/news/south-africa/2020-05-23-group-of-leading-scientists-come-out-in-support-of-glenda-gray-who-dared-to-criticise-lockdown-regulations/.
21 Mark Heywood, 'Malnutrition, Health Services and Democracy: The Responsibility to Speak Out', *Daily Maverick*, 26 May 2020, https://www.dailymaverick.co.za/article/2020-05-26-malnutrition-health-services-and-democracy-the-responsibility-to-speak-out/.
22 News24, 'Glenda Gray "Grateful for Support" as SAMRC Calls off Investigation into Her Lockdown Criticism', 26 May 2020, https://www.news24.com/news24/SouthAfrica/News/glenda-gray-grateful-for-support-as-samrc-calls-off-investigation-into-her-lockdown-criticism-20200526.
23 Katharine Child, 'Society Newsmaker of the Year: Glenda Gray', *Business Live*, 17 December 2020, https://www.businesslive.co.za/fm/features/cover-story/2020-12-17-society-newsmaker-of-the-year-glenda-gray/.
24 Steven Friedman, 'Speaking Power's Truth: South African Media in the Service of the Suburbs', in *Media and Citizenship: Between Marginalisation and Participation*, eds Anthea Garman and Herman Wasserman (Cape Town: HSRC Press, 2017).
25 Matthew Savides, 'Government "Ignored Expert Advice against Exceeding 70% Taxi Capacity"', *Times Live*, 27 August 2020, https://www.timeslive.co.za/news/south-africa/2020-08-27-government-ignored-expert-advice-against-exceeding-70-taxi-capacity.

26   Nonkululeko Njilo, '35 Children Have Died of Covid-19 in Gauteng as Hospital Admissions Drop', *Times Live*, 10 September 2020, https://www.timeslive.co.za/news/south-africa/2020-09-10-35-children-have-died-of-covid-19-in-gauteng-as-hospital-admissions-drop/.
27   William Hanague, 'There Have Been Many Failures over Covid. We Cannot Afford to Forget Them', *The Guardian*, 23 March 2021, https://www.theguardian.com/commentisfree/2021/mar/22/covid-failures-uk-death-rate-pandemic.
28   Adam Habib, *Rebels and Rage: Reflecting on #Fees Must Fall* (Johannesburg: Jonathan Ball, 2019).
29   Friedman, 'Speaking Power's Truth'.
30   BBC, 'Covid-19: Virus "Success" Taiwan to Keep Restrictions despite Vaccine', 11 December 2020, https://www.bbc.com/news/world-asia-55269729.
31   Karim, 'Trends and Next Steps', Slide 25; Elliot Smith, 'South Africa Extends Lockdown but Offers Roadmap for Reopening', *CNBC*, 15 April 2020, https://www.cnbc.com/2020/04/15/south-africa-extends-lockdown-but-offers-roadmap-for-reopening.html.
32   Zintle Mahlati, '2 270 New Covid-19 Cases, but Prof Abdool Karim Assures SA Not in a Second Wave Right Now', *Independent Online*, 22 November 2020, https://www.iol.co.za/news/south-africa/eastern-cape/2-270-new-covid-19-cases-but-prof-abdool-karim-assures-sa-not-in-a-second-wave-right-now-953a696e-5d3b-4c35-b73c-91bc3ffb0d5b.
33   Sihle Mlambo, 'Coronavirus Will Affect 60–70% of South Africans, Warns Mkhize', *Independent Online*, 20 March 2020, https://www.iol.co.za/news/south-africa/gauteng/coronavirus-will-affect-60-70-of-south-africans-warns-mkhize-45259076.
34   Mlambo, 'Coronavirus'.
35   James C. Scott, *Seeing Like a State: How Certain Schemes to Improve the Human Condition Have Failed* (New Haven, CT: Yale University Press, 1998), 11.
36   Steven Friedman, 'Government's Covid-19 Science Mask Is Slipping', *New Frame*, 8 May 2020, https://www.newframe.com/governments-covid-19-science-mask-is-slipping/.
37   South African Government, 'President Cyril Ramaphosa: Developments in South Africa's Risk-Adjusted Strategy to Manage the Spread of Coronavirus Covid-19', 24 May 2020, https://www.gov.za/speeches/president-cyril-ramaphosa-developments-south-africa%E2%80%99s-risk-adjusted-strategy-manage-spread.
38   Business for South Africa, 'Covid 19', https://www.businessforsa.org/business-for-sa-update-and-support-for-lockdown-extension/.
39   Yudelman, 'The Emergence of Modern South Africa'.
40   Business for South Africa, 'Covid 19'.
41   Khulekani Magubane and Lameez Omarjee, 'Covid-19: Govt's Economic Rescue Plan a Race against Time', *Fin24*, 19 April 2020, https://www.news24.com/fin24/economy/south-africa/covid-19-govts-economic-rescue-plan-a-race-against-time-20200419.
42   Carol Paton, 'Business for SA Urges Urgent Opening of Economy to Avoid Jobs Bloodbath', *Business Live*, 6 May 2020, https://www.businesslive.co.za/

bd/national/2020-05-06-business-for-sa-urges-urgent-opening-of-economy-to-avoid-jobs-bloodbath/.
43 Lukanyo Myanda, 'Government May be Seeing the Light on Need to Open Economy, Says Cas Coovadia', *Business Live*, 20 May 2020, https://www.businesslive.co.za/bd/economy/2020-05-20-government-may-be-seeing-the-light-on-need-to-open-economy-says-cas-coovadia/.
44 Sergio Correia, Stephan Luck and Emil Verner, 'Pandemics Depress the Economy, Public Health Interventions Do Not: Evidence from the 1918 Flu', 11 June 2020, https://ssrn.com/abstract=3561560 or http://dx.doi.org/10.2139/ssrn.3561560.
45 International Monetary Fund, 'World Economic Outlook, October 2020: A Long and Difficult Ascent', https://www.imf.org/en/Publications/WEO/Issues/2020/09/30/world-economic-outlook-october-2020, p.64.
46 South African Government, 'Coronavirus Covid-19 Alert Level 1', https://www.gov.za/covid-19/about/coronavirus-covid-19-alert-level-1#.
47 Lizeka Tandwa and Qaanita Hunter, 'Lockdown: Ramaphosa Lobbied to Open Places of Worship', *News24*, 21 May 2020, https://www.news24.com/news24/SouthAfrica/News/lockdown-ramaphosa-lobbied-to-open-places-of-worship-20200521.
48 South African Government News Agency, 'Places of Worship to Resume Services under Level 3 of Lockdown', 26 May 2020, https://www.sanews.gov.za/south-africa/places-worship-resume-services-under-level-3-lockdown.
49 Nelisiwe Msomi, 'During the Covid-19 Pandemic, Religious Leaders Build Resilience', *Health-e News*, 12 June 2020, https://health-e.org.za/2020/06/12/during-the-covid-19-pandemic-religious-leaders-build-resilience/.
50 Phillip de Wet, 'A Third of SA's Golf Clubs May Not Survive Lockdown – Here's How They Hope to Open Sooner', *Business Insider SA*, 29 April 2020, https://www.businessinsider.co.za/golf-course-plans-to-return-under-south-africas-lockdown-as-healthy-exercise-2020-4.
51 Government Communication and Information Service (GCIS), 'Level 3 Lockdown: New Regulations for Arts and Cultural Spaces', 7 July 2020, https://www.enca.com/news/sa-lockdown-mthethwa-announces-new-regulations-reopening-cinemas-and-sport.
52 Craig Ray, 'Level 3 Regulations Edge SA Sports Federations to the Brink', *Daily Maverick*, 1 June 2020, https://www.dailymaverick.co.za/article/2020-06-01-level-3-regulations-edge-sa-sports-federations-to-the-brink/.
53 Mkhize, 'Slideshow'.
54 South African Government News Agency, 'SA Moves to Level 3 of Lockdown', 28 December 2020, https://www.sanews.gov.za/south-africa/sa-moves-level-3-lockdown.
55 Laura Gamba, 'Latin America Begins Reopening as Virus Cases Rise', *AA*, 2 June 2020, https://www.aa.com.tr/en/americas/latin-america-begins-reopening-as-virus-cases-rise/1861492.
56 Smith, 'South Africa Extends Lockdown'.
57 Marelise van der Merwe, 'Some Businesses Will Reopen in May – but it Won't be Business as Usual', *Fin24*, 23 April 2020, https://www.news24.

58 com/fin24/economy/south-africa/some-businesses-will-reopen-but-it-wont-be-business-as-usual-20200423.
58 Calculated using official figures available at https://sacoronavirus.co.za.
59 TimesLive, 'Business Travel to be Phased in under Level 3 – President Cyril Ramaphosa', 24 May 2020, https://www.timeslive.co.za/politics/2020-05-24-business-travel-to-be-phased-in-under-level-3-president-cyril-ramaphosa/.
60 Calculated using official figures available at https://sacoronavirus.co.za.
61 Calculated using official figures available at https://sacoronavirus.co.za.
62 Karim, 'Trends and Next Steps', Slide 10.
63 Neva Makgetla, with Lutendo Maiwashe, *TIPS Tracker: The Economy and the Pandemic* (Tshwane: Trade and Industry Policy Strategies, 2020).
64 Edwin Ntshidi, 'Gauteng Taxi Drivers Violate Lockdown Rules despite Law Enforcement Presence', *Eyewitness News*, 29 June 2020, https://ewn.co.za/2020/06/29/gauteng-taxi-drivers-violate-lockdown-rules-despite-law-enforcement-presence.
65 Ray White, 'Mbalula: Government Won't Tolerate Breaking of Lockdown Rules by Taxi Industry', *Eyewitness News*, 16 July 2020, https://ewn.co.za/2020/07/16/govt-won-t-tolerate-breaking-of-lockdown-rules-by-taxi-industry-says-mbalula.
66 Azarrah Karrim, 'Parents, Cosas Join Forces to Stop Govt's "Irrational" Reopening of Schools', *News24*, 23 May 2020, https://www.news24.com/news24/southafrica/news/parents-cosas-join-forces-to-stop-govts-irrational-reopening-of-schools-20200523.
67 Nonkululeko Njilo, '53% of Adults Want Schools Closed until Covid-19 Situation Improves – Survey', *Times Live*, 13 January 2021, https://www.timeslive.co.za/news/south-africa/2021-01-13-53-of-adults-want-schools-closed-until-covid-19-situation-improves-survey/.
68 Brian W. Simpson, 'The Important and Elusive Science behind Safely Reopening Schools', Johns Hopkins Bloomberg School of Public Health, 14 August 2020, https://www.jhsph.edu/covid-19/articles/the-important-and-elusive-science-behind-safely-reopening-schools.html.
69 Steven Friedman, 'The Forgotten Sovereign: Citizens, States and Foreign Policy in the South', in *Diplomacy and Developing Nations: Post-Cold War Foreign Policy-Making Structures and Processes*, eds Justin Robertson and Maurice A. East (Abingdon: Routledge, (2005), 225–252.
70 Steven Friedman and Mark Robinson, 'Civil Society, Democratization, and Foreign Aid: Civic Engagement and Public Policy in South Africa and Uganda', *Democratization* 14, no. 4 (2007): 643–668.
71 Redaction Africanews, 'Protests Erupt in Senegal over New Covid-19 Measures', *Africanews*, 7 January 2021, https://www.africanews.com/2021/01/07/protests-erupt-in-senegal-over-new-covid-19-measures/.
72 Khumalo, 'South Africans Are Now Gatvol'.
73 Zakhele Mthembu, 'ANC Followed Chinese Communist Party Playbook in Lockdown, Sacrificing Our Freedom', *City Press*, 22 December 2020, https://www.news24.com/citypress/voices/anc-followed-chinese-communist-party-playbook-in-lockdown-sacrificing-our-freedom-20201221.

Notes

CHAPTER 4: The Blank Cheque

1   Peter Newell, 'Taking Accountability into Account: The Debate so Far', in *Rights, Resources and the Politics of Accountability*, eds Peter Newell and Joanna Wheeler (London: Zed Books, 2006), 37–58.
2   Steven Friedman and Omano Edigheji, *Eternal (and Internal) Tensions? Conceptualising Public Accountability in South African Higher Education* (Pretoria: Council on Higher Education, December 2006).
3   Steven Friedman, 'Archipelagos of Dominance: Party Fiefdoms and South African Democracy', *Zeitschrift für Vergleichende Politikwissenschaft (Journal of Comparative Politics)* 9, no. 3 (2015): 139–159.
4   Fin24, 'SARB: Unsecured Lending on the Rise', 28 June 2013, http://www.fin24.com/ Debt/News/Sarb-Unsecured-lending-on-the-rise-20130628.
5   Edward Webster, 'The Promise and the Possibility: South Africa's Contested Industrial Relations Path', *Transformation* 81/82 (2013): 208–235.
6   The Human Sciences Research Council's 2017 Social Attitudes Survey contained a section on 'Financial Literacy' which discussed, among other issues, the lack of a 'savings mentality' among South Africans. This of course assumes that people don't save because they lack the right attitude, not because they may not be able to afford saving. Benjamin Roberts, Jare Struwig, Steven Gordon and Thobeka Radebe, 'Financial Literacy in South Africa', Results from the 2017/18 South African Social Attitudes Survey round, report prepared by the Human Sciences Research Council on behalf of the Financial Sector Conduct Authority, Pretoria, 2018.
7   Douglas Gibson, 'Opinion: Unions Must Stop Being Greedy in These Times of Crisis', *The Star*, 15 October 2020, https://www.iol.co.za/the-star/opinion-analysis/opinion-unions-must-stop-being-greedy-in-these-times-of-crisis-e90a5993-f920-46b6-88db-55d3bd513336.
8   Ntwaagae Seleka, 'Covid-19 Spike: Many Private Hospitals Full, Patients Sent to Public Hospitals – Health Minister', *News24*, 29 December 2020, https://www.news24.com/news24/southafrica/news/covid-19-spike-many-private-hospitals-full-patients-sent-to-public-hospitals-health-minister-20201229.
9   Antony Sguazzin and Pauline Bax, 'Where Are Our Coronavirus Vaccines? South Africans Ask', *Bloomberg*, 21 January 2021, https://www.bloomberg.com/news/articles/2021-01-21/south-africa-s-vaccine-holdup-heaps-pressure-on-ramaphosa.
10 South African Department of Health, 'Covid-19 Coronavirus South African Resource Portal', https://sacoronavirus.co.za/.
11 Black Sash Western Cape Region, 'The Coloured Labour Preference Area Policy', Paper presented by Cape Western Region to National Conference, 1983, http://disa.ukzn.ac.za/cnf19830311026001000.
12 Africa News Agency (ANA), 'Cape Town's Covid-19 Spike Occurred in Malls in Last Weeks of Hard Lockdown: Prof Karim', *Independent Online*, 29 May 2020, https://www.iol.co.za/news/south-africa/western-cape/cape-towns-covid-19-spike-occurred-in-malls-in-last-weeks-of-hard-lockdown-prof-karim-48691940.

13 Daniel Uys and Schalk van der Merwe, 'Why Is the Covid-19 Mortality Rate so High in the Western Cape?' *Business Live*, 2 July 2020, https://www.businesslive.co.za/bd/opinion/2020-07-02-why-is-the-covid-19-mortality-rate-so-high-in-the-western-cape/.
14 Alice Street, *Biomedicine in an Unstable Place: Infrastructure and Personhood in a Papua New Guinean Hospital* (Durham, NC: Duke University Press, 2014).
15 Marcus Low, 'SA Doctors Concerned about Severe Covid-19 Testing Delays', *Daily Maverick*, 8 May 2020, https://www.dailymaverick.co.za/article/2020-05-08-sa-doctors-concerned-about-severe-covid-19-testing-delays/.
16 Liezl Human, 'Huge Delays in Covid-19 Test Results', *GroundUp*, 8 May 2020, https://www.groundup.org.za/article/huge-delays-covid-19-test-results/.
17 Parliamentary Monitoring Group, 'NHLS Strategy to Deal with Covid-19 Test Results and Backlogs; Life Healthcare Group & Netcare on State of Readiness for Covid-19', https://pmg.org.za/page/NHLSstrategytodealwithCovid19testresultsandbacklogs.
18 Katharine Child, 'SA Needn't Fear the "Second Wave", Says Madhi', *Business Live*, 14 September 2020, https://www.businesslive.co.za/fm/features/2020-09-14-sa-neednt-fear-the-second-wave-says-madhi/.
19 Shabir A. Madhi, 'South Africa Failed to Get its Act Together on Vaccines: Here's How', *The Conversation*, 15 January 2021, https://heconversation.com/south-africa-failed-to-get-its-act-together-on-vaccines-heres-how-153384.
20 Gauteng Visual Analytics Platform, https://gpcoronavirus.co.za/#hotspots.
21 Bank, 'Ground Zero'.
22 South African Broadcasting Corporation (SABC), 'Tembisa Hospital CEO to Face Suspension after Patient's Untimely Death', 30 January 2021, https://www.sabcnews.com/sabcnews/tembisa-hospital-ceo-to-face-suspension-after-patients-untimely-death/.
23 Laila Majiet, 'How Covid-19 Advanced Gauteng Critical Care by up to 20 Years', *Power 98.7*, 29 January 2021, https://www.power987.co.za/news/how-covid-19-advanced-gauteng-critical-care-by-up-to-20-years/.
24 National Institute for Communicable Diseases, 'Latest Confirmed Cases of Covid-19 in South Africa, 29 January 2021', https://www.nicd.ac.za/latest-confirmed-cases-of-covid-19-in-south-africa-29-jan-2021/.
25 Sihle Mlambo, 'Covid-19 ICU Mortality Reduced by 25% since Introduction of Dexamethasone', *Independent Online*, 5 August 2020, https://www.iol.co.za/news/south-africa/covid-19-icu-mortality-reduced-by-25-since-introduction-of-dexamethasone-0c7fa57e-f00b-47b5-bbe9-1fa21435e3e7.
26 Staff Writer, 'Over 106,000 Excess Deaths Reported in South Africa since First Covid-19 Wave', *BusinessTech*, 25 January 2021, https://businesstech.co.za/news/trending/463168/over-106000-excess-deaths-reported-in-south-africa-since-first-covid-19-wave/.
27 Steven Friedman, 'A New Menace Is Stalking the Land, Yet No One Is Talking about it', *Business Day*, 26 January 2021, https://www.businesslive.co.za/bd/opinion/columnists/2021-01-26-steven-friedman-a-new-menace-is-stalking-the-land-yet-no-one-is-talking-about-it/.
28 Machanik, 'Free the Evidence'.

29 Brent Lindeque, 'Groote Schuur Hospital Celebrates 150 Ventilator Survivor', *Good Things Guy*, 2 March 2021, https://www.goodthingsguy.com/business/groote-schuur-hospital-celebrates-150-ventilator-survivor/.
30 Anthula Higgins, 'State Must "Get out the Way" of Economic Recovery', Democratic Alliance, 2 October 2020, https://content.voteda.org/blog/2020/10/state-must-get-out-the-way-of-economic-recovery/.
31 Citizen reporter, 'Twitter Reacts: ANC Calls out Police Brutality in the US, but What about Collins Khosa?' *The Citizen*, 2 June 2020, https://citizen.co.za/news/south-africa/social-media/2295368/twitter-reacts-anc-calls-out-police-brutality-in-the-us-but-what-about-collins-khosa/.
32 Hyonhee Shin, 'South Korea to Tighten Social Distancing, Warns of New Covid-19 Crisis', *Reuters*, 17 November 2020, https://www.reuters.com/article/us-health-coronavirus-southkorea-idUSKBN27W32M.
33 New Zealand Herald, 'Covid-19 Coronavirus: Auckland in Alert Level 3 Lockdown for a Week, Rest of NZ at Level 2 – Jacinda Ardern', *New Zealand Herald*, 27 February 2021, https://www.nzherald.co.nz/nz/covid-19-coronavirus-auckland-in-alert-level-3-lockdown-for-a-week-rest-of-nz-at-level-2-jacinda-ardern/OWBIIXGYZQIPJL36WZYZKSEWH4/.
34 Madhi, 'South Africa Failed'; eNCA, 'Dr Aslam Dasoo: Govt Dropped the Ball in Securing Covid-19 Vaccine', 3 January 2021, https://www.enca.com/news/dr-aslam-dasoo-govt-dropped-ball-securing-covid-19-vaccine.
35 Tebogo Monama, 'Vaccination Hubs Conduct Dry Runs as They Wait for Johnson & Johnson Vaccine to Land', *News24*, 16 February 2021, https://www.news24.com/news24/southafrica/news/vaccination-hubs-conduct-dry-runs-as-they-wait-for-johnson-johnson-vaccine-to-land-20210216.
36 eNCA, 'The Benefits Outweigh the Risks: Prof Madhi on J&J Vaccine', 15 April 2021, https://www.enca.com/news/benefits-outweigh-risks-prof-madhi-jj-vaccine.
37 John Steenhuisen, 'Vaccination Must Replace Lockdown if SA Is to Survive Covid-19', Democratic Alliance, 28 December 2020, https://www.da.org.za/2020/12/vaccination-must-replace-lockdown-if-sa-is-to-survive-covid-19.
38 Sam Meredith, 'Chile Has One of the World's Best Vaccination Rates. Covid Is Surging There Anyway', *CNBC*, 19 April 2021, https://www.cnbc.com/2021/04/19/covid-chiles-coronavirus-cases-hit-record-levels-despite-vaccine-rollout.html.
39 Kenan Malik, 'Coronavirus Vaccines Offer the World Hope – Unless You Live in Africa', *The Guardian*, 24 January 2021, https://www.theguardian.com/commentisfree/2021/jan/24/coronavirus-vaccines-offer-the-world-hope-unless-you-live-in-africa.
40 This argument is a modified repetition of that made in Steven Friedman, 'The Public Debate: A Cure Worse than the Disease', Democracy Development Programme, 15 February 2021, https://ddp.org.za/blog/2021/02/15/the-public-debate-a-cure-worse-than-the-disease/.
41 Peter Bruce, 'Hello, Useless ANC. I Phoned Moderna and They Have Vaccines for Us', *Business Live*, 20 January 2021, https://www.businesslive.co.za/bd/opinion/columnists/2021-01-20-peter-bruce-hello-useless-anc-i-phoned-moderna-and-they-have-vaccines-for-us/.

42   Simone Reperger, 'The Pandemic Cannot be Defeated by Vaccination Alone', *International Politics and Society*, 26 April 2021, https://www.ips-journal.eu/interviews/the-pandemic-cannot-be-defeated-by-vaccination-alone-5142/.
43   Azarrah Karrim, 'Prof Shabir Madhi "Mortified" at Decision on AstraZeneca Vaccine, Says it Might Expire', *News24*, 2 March 2021, https://www.news24.com/news24/southafrica/investigations/covid19/prof-shabir-madhi-mortified-at-decision-on-astrazeneca-vaccine-says-it-might-expire-20210302.
44   Shabir A. Madhi, 'Decision Not to Use Astrazeneca Vaccine Goes against the Spirit of What the Health Department Espoused', *Business Live*, 5 March 2021, https://www.businesslive.co.za/bd/opinion/2021-03-04-shabir-a-madhi-decision-not-to-use-astrazeneca-vaccine-goes-against-the-spirit-of-what-the-health-department-espoused/.
45   Kevin Rawlinson and Ian Sample, 'Oxford Covid Vaccine Has 10% Efficacy against South African Variant, Study Suggests', *The Guardian*, 8 February 2021, https://www.theguardian.com/world/2021/feb/08/oxford-covid-vaccine-10-effective-south-african-variant-study.
46   Barry Schoub, 'The ABC of AstraZeneca Vaccine and the B.1.351 Variant', *News24*, 23 March 2021, https://www.news24.com/news24/analysis/barry-schoub-the-abc-of-astrazeneca-vaccine-and-the-b1351-variant-20210323.
47   Adriaan Basson, 'Lockdown All but Over as Government Shifts to Individual Responsibility', *News24*, 17 June 2020, https://www.news24.com/news24/analysis/first-take-lockdown-all-but-over-as-government-shifts-to-individual-responsibility-20200617.
48   Alan Winde, 'Western Cape Is Planning for 3rd Wave; Personal Responsibility Remains Key', Western Cape Government Covid-19 Response: Let's Stop the Spread, 3 March 2021, https://coronavirus.westerncape.gov.za/news/western-cape-planning-3rd-wave-personal-responsibility-remains-key.
49   Mahlati, '2 270 New Covid-19 Cases'.
50   Malibongwe Dayimani, 'Eastern Cape Health MEC to Target Taverns amid Covid-19 Second Wave Concerns', *News24*, 23 November 2020, https://www.news24.com/news24/southafrica/news/eastern-cape-health-mec-to-target-taverns-amid-covid-19-second-wave-concerns-20201123.
51   The report was titled *Closing the Gate: Death, Dignity and Distress in Rural Eastern Cape in the Time of Covid-19* and was reported in Bank, 'Ground Zero', and Leslie Bank, 'The Sociology of Ground Zero: The South African Variant and Colonial Prejudice', *African Arguments*, 26 February 2021, https://africanarguments.org/2021/02/the-sociology-of-ground-zero-south-african-variant-and-colonial-prejudice/.
52   Dayimani, 'Eastern Cape Health MEC'.
53   Bank, 'Ground Zero'.
54   Bank, 'Ground Zero'.

CHAPTER 5: The Path Not Taken

1 Bank, 'Ground Zero'.
2 Johns Hopkins University Coronavirus Resource Center, 'Covid-19 Map', 2021, https://coronavirus.jhu.edu/map.html.
3 Bank, 'Ground Zero'.
4 Bank, 'Ground Zero'.
5 Spinney, 'The Coronavirus Slayer'.
6 Steven Friedman, 'Getting Better than "World Class": The Challenge of Governing Postapartheid South Africa', *Social Research* 72, no. 3 (Fall 2005): 757–784.
7 Brian Sokutu, 'SA Has to "Learn from Asian Tigers" to Move Economy', *The Citizen*, 29 August 2019, https://citizen.co.za/business/business-news/2172592/sa-has-to-learn-from-asian-tigers-to-move-economy/.
8 Zweli Mkhize, 'Welcoming Remarks at Arrival of World Health Organisation Officials to Assist in Coronavirus Covid-19 Pandemic', South African Government, 14 August 2020, https://www.gov.za/speeches/minister-zweli-mkhize-welcoming-remarks-arrival-world-health-organisation-officials-assist#.
9 Bernault, 'Some Lessons'.
10 Seleka, 'Covid-19 Spike'.
11 John Kent, 'Thousands Have Been Refused Funding to Self-Isolate. No Wonder Covid Is Rampant', *The Guardian*, 22 January 2021, https://www.theguardian.com/commentisfree/2021/jan/22/funding-self-isolate-covid-rampant.
12 South African Government, 'Minister Tito Mboweni: 2021 Budget Speech', 24 February 2021, https://www.gov.za/speeches/minister-tito-mboweni-2021-budget-speech-24-feb-2021-0000.
13 South African Government, 'Zola Sidney Themba Skweyiya, Dr', https://www.gov.za/about-government/contact-directory/zola-sidney-themba-skweyiya-dr.
14 Staff Writer, 'How Many South Africans Now Rely on Social Grants: 1996 vs 2020', *Businesstech*, 10 January 2021, https://businesstech.co.za/news/government/459186/how-many-south-africans-now-rely-on-social-grants-1996-vs-2020/.
15 Steven Friedman, 'The More Things Change … South Africa's Democracy and the Burden of the Past', *Social Research* 86, no. 1 (Spring 2019): 279–303.
16 The Lancet, 'Editorial: Covid-19 in Latin America: A Humanitarian Crisis', *The Lancet* 396, no. 10261 (2020): 1, https://doi.org/10.1016/S0140-6736(20)32328-X.
17 Guillermo O' Donnell, 'Illusions about Consolidation', *Journal of Democracy* 7, no. 2 (April 1996): 34–51.

REFERENCES

Secondary sources

Aschwanden, Christie. 'The False Promise of Herd Immunity for Covid-19'. *Nature*, 21 October 2020. https://www.nature.com/articles/d41586-020-4:02948-4.

Bernault, Florence. 'Some Lessons from the History of Epidemics in Africa'. *African Arguments*, 6 June 2020. https://africanarguments.org/2020/06/some-lessons-from-the-history-of-epidemics-in-africa/.

Bhorat, Haroon, Aalia Cassim and Alan Hirsch. *Policy Co-ordination and Growth Traps in a Middle-Income Country Setting: The Case of South Africa*. WIDER Working Paper 2014/155. Helsinki, United Nations University World Institute for Development Economics Research, 2014.

Black Sash Western Cape Region. 'The Coloured Labour Preference Area Policy'. Paper presented by Cape Western Region to National Conference, 11 March 1983. http://disa.ukzn.ac.za/cnf19830311026001000.

Bräutigam, Deborah. 'Contingent Consent: Export Taxation and State Building in Mauritius'. Paper presented at the annual meeting of the American Political Science Association, Marriott, Loews Philadelphia, and the Pennsylvania Convention Center, Philadelphia, PA, 31 August 2006.

Correia, Sergio, Stephan Luck and Emil Verner. 'Pandemics Depress the Economy, Public Health Interventions Do Not: Evidence from the 1918 Flu (June 5)'. 2020. https://ssrn.com/abstract=3561560 or http://dx.doi.org/10.2139/ssrn.3561560.

Friedman, Steven. 'The Forgotten Sovereign: Citizens, States and Foreign Policy in the South'. In *Diplomacy and Developing Nations: Post-Cold War Foreign Policy-Making Structures and Processes*, edited by Justin Robertson and Maurice A. East, pp. 225–252. Abingdon: Routledge, 2005.

Friedman, Steven. 'Getting Better than "World Class": The Challenge of Governing Postapartheid South Africa'. *Social Research* 72, no. 3 (Fall 2005): 757–784.

Friedman, Steven. 'Gaining Comprehensive AIDS Treatment in South Africa: The Extraordinary "Ordinary"'. In *Citizen Action and National Policy Reform*, edited by John Gaventa and Rosemary McGee, 44–68. London: Zed Books, 2010.

Friedman, Steven. 'Seeing Ourselves as Others See Us: Racism, Technique and the Mbeki Administration'. In *Mbeki and After: Reflections on the Legacy of Thabo*

Mbeki, edited by Daryl Glaser, 163–186. Johannesburg: Wits University Press, 2010.

Friedman, Steven. 'Archipelagos of Dominance. Party Fiefdoms and South African Democracy'. *Zeitschrift für Vergleichende Politikwissenschaft (Journal of Comparative Politics)* 9, no. 3 (2015): 139–159.

Friedman, Steven. 'Speaking Power's Truth: South African Media in the Service of the Suburbs'. In *Media and Citizenship: Between Marginalisation and Participation*, edited by Anthea Garman and Herman Wasserman. Cape Town: HSRC Press, 2017.

Friedman, Steven. 'The More Things Change … South Africa's Democracy and the Burden of the Past'. *Social Research* 86, no. 1 (Spring 2019): 279–303.

Friedman, Steven. *Prisoners of the Past: South African Democracy and the Legacy of Minority Rule.* Johannesburg: Wits University Press, 2021.

Friedman, Steven and Omano Edigheji. *Eternal (and Internal) Tensions? Conceptualising Public Accountability in South African Higher Education.* Pretoria: Council on Higher Education, 2006.

Friedman, Steven and Mark Robinson. 'Civil Society, Democratization, and Foreign Aid: Civic Engagement and Public Policy in South Africa and Uganda'. *Democratization* 14, no. 4 (2007): 643–668.

Friedman, Steven and Zimitri Erasmus. 'Counting on "Race": What the Surveys Say (and Do Not Say) about "Race" and Redress'. In *Racial Redress and Citizenship in South Africa*, edited by Adam Habib and Kristina Bentley, 33–74. Cape Town: HSRC Press, 2008.

Geffen, Nathan. *Echoes of Lysenko: State-Sponsored Pseudo-Science in South Africa.* CSSR Working Paper No. 149. Cape Town, Centre for Social Science Research, Aids and Society Research Unit, March 2006.

Giliomee, Hermann. 'An Extraordinary Country'. In *The Last Afrikaner Leaders: A Supreme Test of Power*, 17–37. Charlottesville: University of Virginia Press, 2012.

Habib, Adam. *Rebels and Rage: Reflecting on #Fees Must Fall.* Johannesburg: Jonathan Ball, 2019.

Heneghan, Carl, Jon Brassey and Tom Jefferson. 'Covid-19: What Proportion Are Asymptomatic?' The Centre for Evidence-Based Medicine, Oxford University, 6 April 2020. https://www.cebm.net/covid-19/covid-19-what-proportion-are-asymptomatic/.

Hotez, Peter. 'Anti-Science Kills: From Soviet Embrace of Pseudoscience to Accelerated Attacks on US Biomedicine'. *PLoS Biol* 19, no. 1 (2021): e3001068. https://doi.org/10.1371/journal.pbio.3001068.

Humphries, Richard, Thabo Rapoo and Steven Friedman. 'The Shape of the Country: Negotiating Regional Government'. In *The Small Miracle: South Africa's Negotiated Settlement*, edited by Steven Friedman and Doreen Atkinson, 148–181. Johannesburg: Ravan Press, 1994.

International Monetary Fund. 'World Economic Outlook, October 2020: A Long and Difficult Ascent'. 2020. https://www.imf.org/en/Publications/WEO/Issues/2020/09/30/world-economic-outlook-october-2020.

Khan Burki, Talha. 'Herd Immunity for Covid-19'. *The Lancet Respiratory Medicine* 9, no. 2 (November 2020): 135–136.

The Lancet. 'Editorial: Covid-19 in Latin America: A Humanitarian Crisis'. *The Lancet* 396, no. 10261 (2020): 1. https://doi.org/10.1016/S0140-6736(20)32328-X.

Logue, Jennifer K., Nicholas M. Franko, Denise J. McCulloch et al. 'Sequelae in Adults at 6 Months after Covid-19 Infection'. *JAMA Network Open* 4, no. 2 (2021): e210830. doi:10.1001/jamanetworkopen.2021.0830.

Makgetla, Neva with Lutendo Maiwashe. *TIPS Tracker: The Economy and the Pandemic*. Tshwane, Trade and Industry Policy Strategies, 2020.

Matthews, Owen. 'Britain Drops Its Go-It-Alone Approach to Coronavirus'. *Foreign Policy*, 17 March 2020. https://foreignpolicy.com/2020/03/17/britain-uk-coronavirus-response-johnson-drops-go-it-alone/.

Mbali, Mandisa. 'Mbeki's Denialism and the Ghosts of Apartheid and Colonialism for Post-Apartheid AIDS Policy-Making'. Workshop paper presented at University of Natal, School of Development Studies, Durban, 15 April 2002. www.hivan.org.za/admin/documents/Mbeki's20%denialism.doc.

Mendelson, Marc and Shabir Madhi. 'South Africa's Coronavirus Testing Strategy Is Broken and Not Fit for Purpose: It's Time for a Change'. *South African Medical Journal* 110, no. 6 (June 2020): 429–431.

Moodie, T. Dunbar. *The Rise of Afrikanerdom: Power, Apartheid and Afrikaner Civil Religion*. Berkeley: University of California Press, 1980.

Moulder, James. 'The Predominantly White Universities: Some Ideas for a Debate'. In *Knowledge and Power in South Africa*, edited by Jonathan Jansen, 117, 118.. Johannesburg: Skotaville, 1991.

Newell, Peter. 'Taking Accountability into Account: The Debate so Far'. In *Rights, Resources and the Politics of Accountability*, edited by Peter Newell and Joanna Wheeler, 37–58. London: Zed Books, 2006.

Nordling, Linda. '"Our Epidemic Could Exceed a Million Cases" – South Africa's Top Coronavirus Adviser'. *Nature*, 24 July 2020.

Nymanjoh, Anye. 'The Phenomenology of *Rhodes Must Fall*: Student Activism and the Experience of Alienation at the University of Cape Town'. *Strategic Review for Southern Africa* 39, no. 1 (May 2017): 256–277.

O'Donnell, Guillermo. 'Illusions About Consolidation'. *Journal of Democracy* 7, no. 2 (April 1996): 34–51.

Palaniappan, Ashwin, Udit Dave and Brandon Gosine. 'Comparing South Korea and Italy's Healthcare Systems and Initiatives to Combat Covid-19'. *Pan American Journal of Public Health* 44 (2020): e53. https://doi.org/10.26633/RPSP.2020.53.

Parker, Alexandra, Gillian Maree, Graeme Gotz and Samkelisiwe Khanyile. *Women and Covid-19 in Gauteng*. August 2020 Map of the Month, Gauteng City-Region Observatory, 1 September 2020.

Patel, Leila, Yolanda Sadie, Victoria Graham, Aislinn Delaney and Kim Baldry. *Voting Behaviour and the Influence of Social Protection: A Study of Voting Behaviour in Three Poor Areas of South Africa*. Johannesburg: Centre for Social Development in Africa and Department of Politics, University of Johannesburg, June 2014.

Piketty, Thomas. *Capital in the Twenty-First Century*. Cambridge, MA: Harvard University Press, 2014.

Reperger, Simone. 'The Pandemic Cannot be Defeated by Vaccination Alone'. *International Politics and Society*, 26 April 2021. https://www.ips-journal.eu/interviews/the-pandemic-cannot-be-defeated-by-vaccination-alone-5142/.

Roberts, Benjamin, Jare Struwig, Steven Gordon and Thobeka Radebe. 'Financial Literacy in South Africa'. Results from the 2017/18 South African Social Attitudes Survey round. Report prepared by the Human Sciences Research Council on behalf of the Financial Sector Conduct Authority. Pretoria: Financial Sector Conduct Authority, 2018.

Scott, James C. *Seeing Like a State: How Certain Schemes to Improve the Human Condition Have Failed*. New Haven, CT: Yale University Press, 1998.

Seleoane, Mandla. 'Resource Flows in Poor Communities: A Reflection on Four Case Studies'. In *Giving & Solidarity: Resource Flows for Poverty Alleviation in South Africa*, edited by Adam Habib and Brij Maharaj, 121–158. Cape Town: HSRC Press, 2008.

Simpson, Brian W. 'The Important and Elusive Science behind Safely Reopening Schools'. Johns Hopkins Bloomberg School of Public Health, 14 August 2020. https://www.jhsph.edu/covid-19/articles/the-important-and-elusive-science-behind-safely-reopening-schools.html.

Singh, Jerome Amir. 'How South Africa's Ministerial Advisory Committee on Covid-19 Can be Optimised'. *South African Medical Journal* 110, no. 6 (May 2020): 439–442.

Staunton, Ciara, Carmen Swanepoel and Melodie Labuschaigne. 'Between a Rock and a Hard Place: Covid-19 and South Africa's Response'. *Journal of Law and the Biosciences* 7, no. 1 (2020): 1–12. doi:10.1093/jlb/lsaa052.

Street, Alice. *Biomedicine in an Unstable Place: Infrastructure and Personhood in a Papua New Guinean Hospital*. Durham, NC: Duke University Press, 2014.

Turner, Richard. 'Black Consciousness and White Liberals'. *Reality* (July 1972): 20–21.

Von Holdt, Karl. 'South Africa: The Transition to Violent Democracy'. *Review of African Political Economy* 40, no. 138 (2013): 589–604.

Webster, Edward. 'The Promise and the Possibility: South Africa's Contested Industrial Relations Path'. *Transformation* 81, no. 82 (2013): 208–235.

Yudelman, David. *The Emergence of Modern South Africa: State, Capital and the Incorporation of Organized Labor on the South African Gold Fields, 1902–1939*. Cape Town: David Philip, 1984.

Documents

Abdool Karim, Salim. 'SA's Covid-19 Epidemic: Trends and Next Steps'. Prepared for Minister of Health Zweli Mkhize. Presentation, 13 April 2020.

Africa Check. 'Social Grants in South Africa'. 28 February 2017. https://africacheck.org/fact-checks/factsheets/factsheet-social-grants-south-africa-separating-myth-reality.

African National Congress. 'MYANC: More Jobs, More Decent Jobs'. *2019 Election Manifesto*, 2019. https://www.anc1912.org.za/myanc-more-jobs-more-decent-jobs-httpstcoj1hes0kftg.

References

Amato, Beth. 'Second Wave Severity: What Semi-Saved South Africa?' University of the Witwatersrand, Johannesburg, 2020. https://www.wits.ac.za/news/latest-news/research-news/2021/2021-01/second-wave-severity-what-semi-saved-south-africa.html.

Business for South Africa. 'Covid 19'. 2020. https://www.businessforsa.org/business-for-sa-update-and-support-for-lockdown-extension/.

'Countries in the World by Population (2021)'. https://www.worldometers.info/world-population/population-by-country/.

Department of Health. 'Covid-19 Online Resource and News Portal'. https://sacoronavirus.co.za.

eNCA. 'Dr Aslam Dasoo: Govt Dropped the Ball in Securing Covid-19 Vaccine'. 3 January 2021. https://www.enca.com/news/dr-aslam-dasoo-govt-dropped-ball-securing-covid-19-vaccine.

Gauteng Visual Analytics Platform. https://gpcoronavirus.co.za/#hotspots.

Ghebreyesus, Tedros Adhanom. 'WHO Director-General's Opening Remarks at the Mission Briefing on Covid-19 – 12 March 2020'. World Health Organization, 12 March 2020. https://www.who.int/director-general/speeches/detail/who-director-general-s-opening-remarks-at-the-mission-briefing-on-covid-19—12-march-2020.

Government Communication and Information Service (GCIS). 'Level 3 Lockdown: New Regulations for Arts and Cultural Spaces'. 7 July 2020. https://www.enca.com/news/sa-lockdown-mthethwa-announces-new-regulations-reopening-cinemas-and-sport.

Higgins, Anthula. 'State Must "Get out the Way" of Economic Recovery'. Democratic Alliance, 2 October 2020. https://content.voteda.org/blog/2020/10/state-must-get-out-the-way-of-economic-recovery.

indiaonlinepages.com. 'Population of Kerala 2020'. http://www.indiaonlinepages.com/population/kerala-population.

Ineng. 'List of SADC Countries by Population'. https://ineng.co.za/list-of-sadc-countries-by-population/.

Johns Hopkins University Coronavirus Resource Centre (JHU). 'Covid-19 Dashboard'. https://coronavirus.jhu.edu/map.html.

Johns Hopkins University Coronavirus Resource Centre (JHU). 'Covid-19 Map'. 2021. https://coronavirus.jhu.edu/map.html.

Johns Hopkins University. 'Covid-19 Data Repository by the Center for Systems Science and Engineering (CSSE) at Johns Hopkins University'. https://github.com/CSSEGISandData/COVID-19.

Mkhize, Dr Zwelini. 'Slideshow: South Africa Covid-19 Experiences to Date'. WHO Regional Committee for Africa Meeting: Covid-19 Session, 25 August 2020. https://sacoronavirus.co.za/2020/08/25/slideshow-south-africa-covid-19-experiences-to-date-25th-august-2020/.

Mkhize, Zweli. 'Welcoming Remarks at Arrival of World Health Organisation Officials to Assist in Coronavirus Covid-19 Pandemic'. South African Government, 14 August 2020. https://www.gov.za/speeches/minister-zweli-mkhize-welcoming-remarks-arrival-world-health-organisation-officials-assist#.

National Institute for Communicable Diseases. 'Latest Confirmed Cases of Covid-19 in South Africa (24 Jan 2021)'. 2021. https://www.nicd.ac.za/latest-confirmed-cases-of-covid-19-in-south-africa-24-jan-2021/.

National Institute for Communicable Diseases. 'Latest Confirmed Cases of Covid-19 in South Africa, 29 January 2021'. 2021. https://www.nicd.ac.za/latest-confirmed-cases-of-covid-19-in-south-africa-29-jan-2021.

Parliamentary Monitoring Group. 'NHLS Strategy to Deal with Covid-19 Test Results and Backlogs; Life Healthcare Group & Netcare on State of Readiness for Covid-19'. 2020. https://pmg.org.za/page/NHLSstrategytodealwithCovid19testresultsandbacklogs.

Ramaphosa, Cyril. 'South Africa's Risk Adjusted Strategy to Manage Spread of Coronavirus Covid-19'. South African Government, 15 August 2020. https://www.gov.za/speeches/president-cyril- August 15.

South African Department of Health. 'Covid-19 Coronavirus South African Resource Portal'. https://sacoronavirus.co.za/.

South African Government. 'Coronavirus Covid-19 Alert Level 1'. https://www.gov.za/covid-19/about/coronavirus-covid-19-alert-level-1#.

South African Government. 'Covid-19 Models'. https://www.gov.za/covid-19/models/covid-19-models#.

South African Government. 'Regulations and Guidelines – Coronavirus Covid-19'. 2020. https://www.gov.za/covid-19/resources/regulations-and-guidelines-coronavirus-covid-19?gclid=EAIaIQobChMI1Yr9xZq17wIVEu7tCh0UmQn7EAAYASAAEgIlS_D_BwE#.

South African Government. 'President Cyril Ramaphosa: Developments in South Africa's Risk-Adjusted Strategy to Manage the Spread of Coronavirus Covid-19'. 24 May 2020. https://www.gov.za/speeches/president-cyril-ramaphosa-developments-south-africa%E2%80%99s-risk-adjusted-strategy-manage-spread.

South African Government. 'Minister Tito Mboweni: 2021 Budget Speech'. 24 February 2021. https://www.gov.za/speeches/minister-tito-mboweni-2021-budget-speech-24-feb-2021-0000.

South African Government. 'Zola Sidney Themba Skweyiya, Dr'. https://www.gov.za/about-government/contact-directory/zola-sidney-themba-skweyiya-dr.

South African Government News Agency. 'Places of Worship to Resume Services under Level 3 of Lockdown'. 26 May 2020. https://www.sanews.gov.za/south-africa/places-worship-resume-services-under-level-3-lockdown.

South African Government News Agency. 'SA Moves to Level 3 of Lockdown'. 28 December 2020. http://www.sanews.gov.za/south-africa/sa-moves-level-3-lockdown.

South African Medical Research Council. 'Prof Salim Abdool Karim'. https://www.samrc.ac.za/people/prof-salim-abdool-karim.

South African Medical Research Council (SAMRC). 'Report on Weekly Deaths in South Africa'. https://www.samrc.ac.za/reports/report-weekly-deaths-south-africa.

References

Statista. 'Distribution of Coronavirus (Covid-19) Deaths in South Africa as of November 16, 2020, by Age'. 2020. https://www.statista.com/statistics/1127280/coronavirus-covid-19-deaths-by-age-distribution-south-africa/.

Statista. 'Cumulative Number of Coronavirus (Covid-19) Cases in the Nordic Countries (as of February 2, 2021)'. 2021. https://www.statista.com/statistics/1102257/cumulative-coronavirus-cases-in-the-nordics/.

Statista. 'Cumulative Number of Coronavirus (Covid-19) Deaths in the Nordic Countries (as of February 2, 2021)'. 2021. https://www.statista.com/statistics/1113834/cumulative-coronavirus-deaths-in-the-nordics/.

Statista. 'Coronavirus (Covid-19) Deaths Worldwide per One Million Population as of February 4, 2021, by Country'. 2021. https://www.statista.com/statistics/1104709/coronavirus-deaths-worldwide-per-million-inhabitants/.

Statistics South Africa. 'National Household Travel Survey 2013'. *Statistical Release P0320.* https://www.statssa.gov.za/publications/P0320/P03202013.pdf.

Statistics South Africa. 'Mid-Year Population Estimates 2019'. *Statistical Release P0302,* 29 July 2019.

Statistics South Africa. *'Quarterly Employment Statistics (QES)'. Statistical Release P0277,* September 2020.

Steenhuisen, John. 'Vaccination Must Replace Lockdown if SA Is to Survive Covid-19'. Democratic Alliance, 28 December 2020. https://www.da.org.za/2020/12/vaccination-must-replace-lockdown-if-sa-is-to-survive-covid-19.

Winde, Alan. 'Western Cape Is Planning for 3rd Wave; Personal Responsibility Remains Key'. Western Cape Government Covid-19 Response: Let's Stop the Spread, 3 March 2021. https://coronavirus.westerncape.gov.za/news/western-cape-planning-3rd-wave-personal-responsibility-remains-key.

World Health Organization. 'WHO Coronavirus Disease (Covid-19) Dashboard'. https://covid19.who.int/?gclid=EAIaIQobChMIzJKZ4tGs7QIVjtPtCh04mA8iEAAYASAAEgIVW_D_BwE.

World Health Organization. 'Situation Reports on Covid-19 Outbreak – Sitrep 07, 15 April 2020'. External Situation Report 7. Data as reported by 14 April 2020. https://www.afro.who.int/publications/situation-reports-covid-19-outbreak-sitrep-07-15-april-2020.

World Health Organization Democratic Republic of Congo. 'Building on Ebola Response to Tackle Covid-19 in DRC'. 25 June 2020. https://www.afro.who.int/news/building-ebola-response-tackle-covid-19-drc.

Worldometer. 'Countries Where Covid-19 Has Spread'. 3 December 2020. https://www.worldometers.info/coronavirus/countries-where-coronavirus-has-spread/.

Worldometer. 'Coronavirus'. https://www.worldometers.info/coronavirus.

Worldometer. 'Coronavirus Egypt'. https://www.worldometers.info/coronavirus/country/egypt/.

Worldometer. 'Coronavirus Nigeria'. https://www.worldometers.info/coronavirus/country/nigeria/#:~:text=Nigeria%20Coronavirus%3A%2067%2C557%20Cases%20and%201%2C173%20Deaths%20%2D%20Worldometer.

Media articles

Abdool Karim, Salim. 'Differences of Opinion Vital "to Arriving at the Best Advice": Prof Abdool Karim'. *Sowetan*, 17 May 2020. https://www.sowetanlive.co.za/news/south-africa/2020-05-17-differences-of-opinion-vital-to-arriving-at-the-best-advice-prof-abdool-karim.

Africa News Agency (ANA). 'Cape Town's Covid-19 Spike Occurred in Malls in Last Weeks of Hard Lockdown: Prof Karim'. *Independent Online*, 29 May 2020. https://www.iol.co.za/news/south-africa/western-cape/cape-towns-covid-19-spike-occurred-in-malls-in-last-weeks-of-hard-lockdown-prof-karim-48691940.

Africa News Agency (ANA) Reporter. 'Institute of Race Relations Mulls Joining Lockdown Legal Challenges'. *Independent Online*, 20 May 2020. https://www.iol.co.za/news/politics/institute-of-race-relations-mulls-joining-lockdown-legal-challenges-48232061.

Al Jazeera. 'Coronavirus Cases in Africa Cross Two Million Mark: AU Tally'. 19 November 2020. https://www.aljazeera.com/news/2020/11/19/coronavirus-cases-in-africa-surpass-2-million-reuters-tally.

Bach, Joscha. 'Don't "Flatten the Curve," Squash it!' *Medium*, 14 March 2020. https://medium.com/@joschabach/flattening-the-curve-is-a-deadly-delusion-eea324fe9727.

Bai, Nina. 'Still Confused about Masks? Here's the Science behind How Face Masks Prevent Coronavirus'. *UCFS*, 26 June 2020. https://www.ucsf.edu/news/2020/06/417906/still-confused-about-masks-heres-science-behind-how-face-masks-prevent.

Baker, Aryn. 'What South Africa Can Teach Us as Worldwide Inequality Grows'. *Time*, 2 May 2019. https://time.com/longform/south-africa-unequal-country.

Bank, Leslie. 'Ground Zero: Deep-Seated Colonial-Era Prejudice Fuelled the Pandemic in Rural Eastern Cape'. *Daily Maverick*, 24 February 2021. https://www.dailymaverick.co.za/article/2021-02-24-ground-zero-deep-seated-colonial-era-prejudice-fuelled-the-pandemic-in-rural-eastern-cape/.

Bank, Leslie. 'The Sociology of Ground Zero: The South African Variant and Colonial Prejudice'. *African Arguments*, 26 February 2021. https://africanarguments.org/2021/02/the-sociology-of-ground-zero-south-african-variant-and-colonial-prejudice/.

Baskin, Jeremy. 'The Coming Covid Science Sh*tstorm: Responding to the Great Barrington Declaration'. *Arena Online*, 15 October 2020. https://arena.org.au/the-coming-covid-science-shtstorm-responding-to-the-great-barrington-declaration/.

Basson, Adriaan. 'Lockdown All but over as Government Shifts to Individual Responsibility'. *News24*, 17 June 2020. https://www.news24.com/news24/analysis/first-take-lockdown-all-but-over-as-government-shifts-to-individual-responsibility-20200617.

BBC. 'The Gravedigger's Truth: Hidden Coronavirus Deaths'. 26 July 2020. https://www.bbc.com/news/av/world-africa-53521563.

BBC. 'Covid-19: Virus "Success" Taiwan to Keep Restrictions despite Vaccine'. 11 December 2020. https://www.bbc.com/news/world-asia-55269729.

References

Beaubien, Jason. 'The Country with the World's Worst Inequality Is ...'. National Public Radio, 2 April 2018. https://www.npr.org/sections/goatsandsoda/2018/04/02/598864666/the-country-with-the-worlds-worst-inequality-is.

Berting, Natasha. 'Innovative Handwashing Stations Pop up across Africa'. *What Design Can Do*, 7 May 2020. https://www.whatdesigncando.com/stories/handwashing-stations-africa/.

Bowman, Sam. 'Is Rishi Sunak the Most Dangerous Man in Government?' *The Guardian*, 8 February 2021. https://www.theguardian.com/commentisfree/2021/feb/05/rishi-sunak-government-pandemic-chancellor.

Brandt, Kevin. 'Ramaphosa: Covid-19 Screening Drive Will be Intensive and Far-Reaching'. *Eyewitness News*, 31 March 2020. https://ewn.co.za/2020/03/31/ramaphosa-covid-19-screening-drive-will-be-intensive-and-far-reaching.

Bruce, Peter. 'Hello, Useless ANC. I Phoned Moderna and They Have Vaccines for Us'. *Business Live*, 20 January 2021. https://www.businesslive.co.za/bd/opinion/columnists/2021-01-20-peter-bruce-hello-useless-anc-i-phoned-moderna-and-they-have-vaccines-for-us/.

BusinessTech. 'South Africa's State of Disaster Extended by Another Month'. 14 April 2021. https://businesstech.co.za/news/trending/483119/south-africas-state-of-disaster-extended-by-another-month-2/.

Cha, Sangmi and Rocky Swift. 'Symptomless and Spreading, South Korea Battles Surge in Silent Covid-19 Cases'. *Reuters*, 27 November 2020. https://www.reuters.com/article/us-health-coronavirus-asymptomatic-asia/symptomless-and-spreading-south-korea-battles-surge-in-silent-covid-19-cases-idUSKBN2870LV.

Child, Katharine. 'SA's Covid-19 Models Were "Flawed", Says Former NICD Expert'. *Business Live*, 24 April 2020. https://www.businesslive.co.za/fm/features/2020-04-24-sas-covid-19-models-were-flawed-says-former-nicd-expert/.

Child, Katharine. 'SA Needn't Fear the "Second Wave", Says Madhi'. *Business Live*, 14 September 2020. https://www.businesslive.co.za/fm/features/2020-09-14-sa-neednt-fear-the-second-wave-says-madhi/.

Child, Katharine. '"It's a Virus, Not War", Says Dr Aslam Dasoo'. *Business Live*, 1 October 2020. https://www.businesslive.co.za/fm/fm-fox/2020-10-01-profile-its-a-virus-not-war-says-dr-aslam-dasoo.

Child, Katharine. 'Society Newsmaker of the Year: Glenda Gray'. *Business Live*, 17 December 2020. https://www.businesslive.co.za/fm/features/cover-story/2020-12-17-society-newsmaker-of-the-year-glenda-gray/.

Citizen Reporter. 'Twitter Reacts: ANC Calls out Police Brutality in the US, but What about Collins Khosa?' *The Citizen*, 2 June 2020. https://citizen.co.za/news/south-africa/social-media/2295368/twitter-reacts-anc-calls-out-police-brutality-in-the-us-but-what-about-collins-khosa/.

Cohen, Jon. 'South Africa Suspends Use of AstraZeneca's Covid-19 Vaccine after it Fails to Clearly Stop Virus Variant'. *Science*, 8 February 2021. https://www.sciencemag.org/news/2021/02/south-africa-suspends-use-astrazenecas-covid-19-vaccine-after-it-fails-clearly-stop.

Cohut, Maria. '"Ill, Abandoned, Unable to Access Help": Living with Long Covid'. *Medical News Today*, 7 September 2020. https://www.medicalnewstoday.com/articles/ill-abandoned-unable-to-access-help-living-with-long-covid.

Costello, Anthony. 'Poor Support for Self-Isolation Undermines the UK's Covid Vaccination Effort'. *The Guardian*, 10 February 2021. https://www.theguardian.com/commentisfree/2021/feb/10/support-self-isolation-uk-covid-vaccination-effort-virus-replicate-mutations-vaccines.

Daniel, Luke. 'Ramaphosa's Decision to Deploy 73 000 Soldiers Questions Lockdown's End'. *The South African*, 23 April 2020. https://www.thesouthafrican.com/news/does-ramaphosa-sandf-army-deployment-indicate-a-lockdown-extension.

Davis, Rebecca. 'Unpacking the Rationality of South Africa's Lockdown Regulations'. *Daily Maverick*, 14 May 2020. https://www.dailymaverick.co.za/article/2020-05-14-unpacking-the-rationality-of-south-africas-lockdown-regulations/.

Dayimani, Malibongwe. 'Eastern Cape Health MEC to Target Taverns amid Covid-19 Second Wave Concerns'. *News24*, 23 November 2020. https://www.news24.com/news24/southafrica/news/eastern-cape-health-mec-to-target-taverns-amid-covid-19-second-wave-concerns-20201123.

De Wet, Phillip. 'A Third of SA's Golf Clubs May Not Survive Lockdown – Here's How They Hope to Open Sooner'. *Business Insider*, 29 April 2020. https://www.businessinsider.co.za/golf-course-plans-to-return-under-south-africas-lockdown-as-healthy-exercise-2020-4.

Du Plessis, Carien. 'How South Africa's Action on Covid-19 Contrasts Sharply with its Response to AIDS'. *The Guardian*, 27 March 2020. https://www.theguardian.com/global-development/2020/may/27/how-south-africas-action-on-covid-19-contrasts-sharply-with-its-response-to-aids-coronavirus.

Ellis, Estelle. '"Gender-Based Violence Is South Africa's Second Pandemic", Says Ramaphosa.' *Daily Maverick*, 18 June 2020. https://www.dailymaverick.co.za/article/2020-06-18-gender-based-violence-is-south-africas-second-pandemic-says-ramaphosa/.

eNCA. 'Mkhize: Coronavirus May Have Infected Nearly 12m South Africans'. 16 September 2020. https://www.enca.com/news/mkhize-coronavirus-may-have-infected-nearly-12mn-south-africans.

Eyewitness News. 'SAMRC Drops Any Further Investigation into Glenda Gray'. 26 May 2020. https://ewn.co.za/2020/05/26/samrc-drops-any-further-investigation-into-professor-glenda-gray.

Eyewitness News. 'SA Now Has Fifth-Highest Number of Covid-19 Cases in the World'. 20 July 2020. https://ewn.co.za/2020/07/20/sa-now-has-fifth-highest-number-of-covid-19-cases-in-the-world.

Fin24. 'SARB: Unsecured Lending on the Rise'. 28 June 2013. http://www.fin24.com/Debt/News/Sarb-Unsecured-lending-on-the-rise-20130628.

Frellick, Marcia. 'Fauci: "About 40%–45% of Infections Are Asymptomatic"'. *Medscape*, 11 September 2020. https://www.medscape.com/viewarticle/937297.

Friedman, Steven. 'Government's Covid-19 Science Mask Is Slipping'. *New Frame*, 8 May 2020. https://www.newframe.com/governments-covid-19-science-mask-is-slipping/.

Friedman, Steven. 'A New Menace Is Stalking the Land, yet No-One Is Talking About it'. *Business Day*, 26 January 2021. https://www.businesslive.co.za/bd/opinion/columnists/2021-01-26-steven-friedman-a-new-menace-is-stalking-the-land-yet-no-one-is-talking-about-it/.

Friedman, Steven. 'The Public Debate: A Cure Worse than the Disease'. Democracy Development Programme, 15 February 2021. https://ddp.org.za/blog/2021/02/15/the-public-debate-a-cure-worse-than-the-disease/.
Gamba, Laura. 'Latin America Begins Reopening as Virus Cases Rise'. *AA*, 2 June 2020. https://www.aa.com.tr/en/americas/latin-america-begins-reopening-as-virus-cases-rise/1861492.
Gering, Michael and Mojalefa Ralekhetho. 'Walking through the Pandemic Modelling, Exponential Growth and Herd Immunity Maze'. *Daily Maverick*, 8 October 2020. https://www.dailymaverick.co.za/opinionista/2020-10-08-walking-through-the-pandemic-modelling-exponential-growth-and-herd-immunity-maze/.
Gibson, Douglas. 'Unions Must Stop Being Greedy in These Times of Crisis'. *The Star*, 15 October 2020. https://www.iol.co.za/the-star/opinion-analysis/opinion-unions-must-stop-being-greedy-in-these-times-of-crisis-e90a5993-f920-46b6-88db-55d3bd513336.
Greenblo, Allan. 'Social Grant System Has Failed to Uplift South Africans'. *Business Day*, 15 July 2019. https://www.businesslive.co.za/fm/opinion/2019-07-15-allan-greenblo-social-grant-system-has-failed-to-uplift-south-africans/.
Hanague, William. 'There Have Been Many Failures over Covid. We Cannot Afford to Forget Them'. *The Guardian*, 23 March 2021. https://www.theguardian.com/commentisfree/2021/mar/22/covid-failures-uk-death-rate-pandemic.
Harding, Andrew. 'Coronavirus in South Africa: Scientists Explore Surprise Theory for Low Death Rate'. British Broadcasting Corporation, 2 September 2020. https://www.bbc.com/news/world-africa-53998374.
Head, Tom. 'SA's Alcohol Ban Explained: Why Booze Is Barred during Lockdown'. *The South African*, 26 March 2020. https://www.thesouthafrican.com/news/why-alcohol-sale-banned-south-africa-during-lockdown/.
Heywood, Mark. 'Malnutrition, Health Services and Democracy: The Responsibility to Speak Out'. *Daily Maverick*, 26 May 2020. https://www.dailymaverick.co.za/article/2020-05-26-malnutrition-health-services-and-democracy-the-responsibility-to-speak-out/.
Hoecklin, Madeleine. 'Switzerland Nixes AstraZeneca Vaccine until More Evidence Is Obtained. Other EU Countries Rule out Vaccine for Older People'. *Health Policy Watch*, 4 February 2021. https://healthpolicy-watch.news/switzerland-nixes-astrazeneca-vaccine-until-more-evidence-is-obtained-other-eu-countries-rule-out-vaccine-for-older-people/.
Human, Liezl. 'Huge Delays in Covid-19 Test Results'. *GroundUp*, 8 May 2020. https://www.groundup.org.za/article/huge-delays-covid-19-test-results/.
Jacobs, Kirsten. 'Dlamini-Zuma Explains Reasons for Tobacco Ban'. *Cape Town etc.*, 27 May 2020. https://www.capetownetc.com/news/dlamini-zuma-explains-reasons-for-tobacco-ban/.
Jeranji, Tiyese. 'Covid-19: How Mechanical Ventilation Has Saved Lives at Groote Schuur Hospital'. *Spotlight*, 8 September 2020. https://www.spotlightnsp.co.za/2020/09/08/covid-19-how-mechanical-ventilation-has-saved-lives-at-groote-schuur-hospital.
Kahn, Tamar. 'Let More People Go to Work during Lockdown, Institute of Race Relations Urges'. *Business Live*, 2 April 2020. https://www.businesslive.co.za/bd/

national/health/2020-04-02-let-more-people-go-to-work-during-lockdown-institute-of-race-relations-urges.

Kahn, Tamar. 'MRC Board Agrees to Launch Investigation into Glenda Gray'. *Business Live*, 25 May 2020. https://www.businesslive.co.za/bd/national/health/2020-05-25-mrc-board-agrees-to-launch-investigation-into-glenda-gray/.

Karrim, Azarrah. '"I Didn't Criticise the Lockdown, but the Regulations" – Prof Glenda Gray after Mkhize Slams Criticism'. *News24*, 21 May 2020. https://www.news24.com/news24/SouthAfrica/News/i-did-not-criticise-the-lockdown-but-the-regulations-glenda-gray-after-mkhize-slams-criticism-20200521.

Karrim, Azarrah. 'Parents, Cosas Join Forces to Stop Govt's "Irrational" Reopening of Schools'. *News24*, 23 May 2020. https://www.news24.com/news24/southafrica/news/parents-cosas-join-forces-to-stop-govts-irrational-reopening-of-schools-20200523.

Karrim, Azarrah. 'Prof Shabir Madhi "Mortified" at Decision on AstraZeneca Vaccine, Says it Might Expire'. *News24*, 2 March 2021. https://www.news24.com/news24/southafrica/investigations/covid19/prof-shabir-madhi-mortified-at-decision-on-astrazeneca-vaccine-says-it-might-expire-20210302.

Karrim, Azarrah and Sarah Evans. 'Unscientific and Nonsensical: Top Scientist Slams Government's Lockdown Strategy'. *News24*, 16 May 2020. https://www.news24.com/news24/SouthAfrica/News/unscientific-and-nonsensical-top-scientific-adviser-slams-governments-lockdown-strategy-20200516.

Kent, John. 'Thousands Have Been Refused Funding to Self-Isolate. No Wonder Covid Is Rampant'. *The Guardian*, 22 January 2021. https://www.theguardian.com/commentisfree/2021/jan/22/funding-self-isolate-covid-rampant

Khumalo, Juniour. 'South Africans Are Now Gatvol of Lockdown'. *City Press*, 26 April 2020. https://www.news24.com/citypress/Special-Report/Covid-19_Survey/support-for-lockdown-plummets-20200426.

Lehulere, Oupa. 'Scientists against Science: The Campaign to Open "the Economy" in the Time of Covid-19'. *Karibu*, 5 June 2020. https://karibu.org.za/scientists-against-science-the-campaign-to-open-the-economy-in-the-time-of-covid-19/.

Lindeque, Brent. 'Groote Schuur Hospital Celebrates 150 Ventilator Survivor'. *Good Things Guy*, 2 March 2021. https://www.goodthingsguy.com/business/groote-schuur-hospital-celebrates-150-ventilator-survivor/.

Lindeque, Mia. 'SA Can Learn from Europe's Covid-19 Second Wave, Say Experts'. *Eyewitness News*, 3 November 2020. https://ewn.co.za/2020/11/03/sa-can-learn-from-europe-s-covid-19-second-wave-say-experts.

Low, Marcus. 'SA Doctors Concerned about Severe Covid-19 Testing Delays'. *Daily Maverick*, 8 May 2020. https://www.dailymaverick.co.za/article/2020-05-08-sa-doctors-concerned-about-severe-covid-19-testing-delays/.

Low, Marcus and Nathan Geffen. 'Here's What the Models Predict about Covid-19'. *GroundUp*, 22 May 2020. https://www.groundup.org.za/articles/heres-what-models-predict-about-covid19.

Machanik, Philip. 'Covid-19: Free the Evidence'. *Mail & Guardian*, 9 July 2020. https://mg.co.za/coronavirus-essentials/2020-06-09-covid-19-free-the-evidence/.

Madhi, Shabir A. 'South Africa Failed to Get its Act Together on Vaccines: Here's How'. *The Conversation*, 15 January 2021. https://theconversation.com/south-africa-failed-to-get-its-act-together-on-vaccines-heres-how-153384.

Madhi, Shabir A. 'Decision Not to Use AstraZeneca Vaccine Goes against the Spirit of What the Health Department Espoused'. *Business Live*, 5 March 2021. https://www.businesslive.co.za/bd/opinion/2021-03-04-shabir-a-madhi-decision-not-to-use-astrazeneca-vaccine-goes-against-the-spirit-of-what-the-health-department-espoused.

Madhi, Shabir, Alex van den Heever, David Francis, Imraan Valodia, Martin Veller and Michael Sachs. 'South Africa Needs to End the Lockdown: Here's a Blueprint for its Replacement'. *The Conversation*, 9 April 2020. https://theconversation.com/south-africa-needs-to-end-the-lockdown-heres-a-blueprint-for-its-replacement-136080.

Magubane, Khulekani and Lameez Omarjee. 'Covid-19: Govt's Economic Rescue Plan a Race against Time'. *Fin24*, 19 April 2020. https://www.news24.com/fin24/economy/south-africa/covid-19-govts-economic-rescue-plan-a-race-against-time-20200419.

Mahlakoana, Theto. 'Dlamini Zuma's Reasons for Tobacco Sales Plan Are "All Over the Place", Court Hears'. *Eyewitness News*, 10 June 2020. https://ewn.co.za/2020/06/10/dlamini-zuma-s-reasons-for-tobacco-sales-ban-all-over-the-place-court-hears.

Mahlati, Zintle. '2 270 New Covid-19 Cases, but Prof Abdool Karim Assures SA Not in a Second Wave Right Now'. *Independent Online*, 22 November 2020. https://www.iol.co.za/news/south-africa/eastern-cape/2-270-new-covid-19-cases-but-prof-abdool-karim-assures-sa-not-in-a-second-wave-right-now-953a696e-5d3b-4c35-b73c-91bc3ffb0d5b.

Majiet, Laila. 'How Covid-19 Advanced Gauteng Critical Care by up to 20 Years'. *Power 98.7*, 29 January 2021. https://www.power987.co.za/news/how-covid-19-advanced-gauteng-critical-care-by-up-to-20-years/.

Malan, Mia. 'Politicking, Pandemics and Prestige: What's Really behind the Squabbles at South Africa's High-Level Covid-19 Committee?' Bhekisisa Centre for Health Journalism, 19 May 2020. https://bhekisisa.org/article/2020-05-19-ministerial-advisory-committeecommittee-politics-of-science-glenda-gray-salim-abdool-karim-zweli-mkhize.

Malik, Kenan. 'Coronavirus Vaccines Offer the World Hope – unless You Live in Africa'. *The Guardian*, 24 January 2021. https://www.theguardian.com/commentisfree/2021/jan/24/coronavirus-vaccines-offer-the-world-hope-unless-you-live-in-africa.

Malik, Nesrine. 'How Many More Images of Covid Disaster Will it Take to Jolt Rich Countries into Action?' *The Guardian*, 3 May 2021. https://www.theguardian.com/commentisfree/2021/may/03/west-images-covid-disaster-poorer-nations-india-crisisFF.

Malinowski, Susan M. 'Eight Ways to Smash, Not Just Flatten, the Coronavirus Curve'. *Medium*, 2 April 2020.

Matiwane, Zimasa and Paige Muller. 'SA Will Have a Severe Epidemic: Prof Salim Abdool Karim'. *Business Live*, 23 April 2020. https://www.businesslive.co.za/bd/

national/health/2020-04-23-listen-sa-will-have-a-severe-epidemic-prof-salim-abdool-karim/.

Matshiqi, Aubrey. 'Why Manuel Is Right and Wrong about Manyi's "Racism"'. *Business Day*, 8 March 2011. http://www.businessday.co.za/articles/Content.aspx?id=136509.

Medical Xpress. 'Africa Reports "Hopeful" Daily Drop in Coronavirus Cases'. 20 August 2020. https://medicalxpress.com/news/2020-08-africa-daily-coronavirus-cases.html.

Mendelson, Marc and Shabir Madhi. 'South Africa's Covid-19 Testing Strategy Needs Urgent Fixing: Here's How to Do it'. *The Conversation*, 9 May 2020. https://theconversation.com/south-africas-covid-19-testing-strategy-needs-urgent-fixing-heres-how-to-do-it-138225.

Mendenhall, Emily and Andrew Wooyoung Kim. 'People in Soweto Told Us about Their Fears in the First Weeks of South Africa's Lockdown'. *The Conversation*, 8 October 2020. https://theconversation.com/people-in-soweto-told-us-about-their-fears-in-the-first-weeks-of-south-africas-lockdown-142325.

Meredith, Sam. 'Chile Has One of the World's Best Vaccination Rates. Covid Is Surging There Anyway'. *CNBC*, 19 April 2021. https://www.cnbc.com/2021/04/19/covid-chiles-coronavirus-cases-hit-record-levels-despite-vaccine-rollout.html.

Mlambo, Sihle. 'Coronavirus Will Affect 60-70% of South Africans, Warns Mkhize'. *Independent Online*, 20 March 2020. https://www.iol.co.za/news/south-africa/gauteng/coronavirus-will-affect-60-70-of-south-africans-warns-mkhize-45259034.

Mlambo, Sihle. 'Covid-19 ICU Mortality Reduced by 25% since Introduction of Dexamethasone'. *Independent Online*, 5 August 2020. https://www.iol.co.za/news/south-africa/covid-19-icu-mortality-reduced-by-25-since-introduction-of-dexamethasone-0c7fa57e-f00b-47b5-bbe9-1fa21435e3e7.

Mlambo, Sihle. 'SA Nominates Cuban Doctors for Nobel Peace Prize, DA and Action SA Not Pleased'. *Independent Online*, 2 February 2021. https://www.iol.co.za/news/south-africa/gauteng/sa-nominates-cuban-doctors-for-nobel-peace-prize-da-and-action-sa-not-pleased-ca3c8870-1eae-4f89-aa3a-35a9d047d522.

Modise, Kgomotso. 'Patel Explains Why Cooked Food Can't be Sold during Lockdown'. *Eyewitness News*, 21 April 2020. https://ewn.co.za/2020/04/21/patel-explains-why-hot-food-can-t-be-sold-during-lockdown.

Monama, Tebogo. 'Vaccination Hubs Conduct Dry Runs as They Wait for Johnson & Johnson Vaccine to Land'. *News24*, 16 February 2021. https://www.news24.com/news24/southafrica/news/vaccination-hubs-conduct-dry-runs-as-they-wait-for-johnson-johnson-vaccine-to-land-20210216.

Msomi, Nelisiwe. 'During the Covid-19 Pandemic, Religious Leaders Build Resilience'. *Health-e News*, 12 June 2020. https://health-e.org.za/2020/06/12/during-the-covid-19-pandemic-religious-leaders-build-resilience/.

Mthembu, Zakhele. 'ANC Followed Chinese Communist Party Playbook in Lockdown, Sacrificing Our Freedom'. *City Press*, 22 December 2020. https://www.news24.com/citypress/voices/anc-followed-chinese-communist-party-playbook-in-lockdown-sacrificing-our-freedom-20201221.

Mthethwa, Cebelihle. 'South Africa: Coronavirus – Commuters Fear Infection in Overcrowded Taxis, Buses and Trains'. *AllAfrica*, 17 March 2020. https://allafrica.com/stories/202003170127.html.
Munshi, Neil, Joseph Cotterill and Andres Schipani. 'Coronavirus Second Wave Surges across Africa'. *Financial Times*, 17 January 2021. https://www.ft.com/content/3d000093-87a3-48f3-8bb5-4ad9a8316aa1.
Muyingo, Sylvia Kiwuwa. 'Covid-19 Affects Men and Women Differently. It's Important to Track the Data'. *Sowetan*, 6 March 2021. https://www.sowetanlive.co.za/news/south-africa/2021-03-06-covid-19-affects-men-and-women-differently-its-important-to-track-the-data.
Mwai, Peter and Christopher Giles. 'Coronavirus: How Fast Is it Spreading in Africa?' BBC, 17 August 2020.
Myanda, Lukanyo. 'Government May be Seeing the Light on Need to Open Economy, Says Cas Coovadia'. *Business Live*, 20 May 2020. https://www.businesslive.co.za/bd/economy/2020-05-20-government-may-be-seeing-the-light-on-need-to-open-economy-says-cas-coovadia.
Ndlazi, Sakhile. 'Covid-19: Back-to-School Fears Mount'. *Pretoria News*, 29 April 2020. https://www.iol.co.za/pretoria-news/covid-19-back-to-school-fears-mount-47325768.
News24. 'Zweli Mkhize's Statement on Prof Glenda Gray's Criticism of Lockdown Regulations'. 21 May 2020. https://www.news24.com/news24/SouthAfrica/News/read-in-full-zweli-mkhizes-statement-on-prof-glenda-grays-criticism-of-lockdown-regulations-20200521.
News24. 'Glenda Gray "Grateful for Support" as SAMRC Calls off Investigation into Her Lockdown Criticism'. 26 May 2020. https://www.news24.com/news24/SouthAfrica/News/glenda-gray-grateful-for-support-as-samrc-calls-off-investigation-into-her-lockdown-criticism-20200526.
New Zealand Herald. 'Covid-19 Coronavirus: Auckland in Alert Level 3 Lockdown for a Week, Rest of NZ at Level 2 – Jacinda Ardern'. *New Zealand Herald*, 27 February 2021. https://www.nzherald.co.nz/nz/covid-19-coronavirus-auckland-in-alert-level-3.
Njilo, Nonkululeko. '35 Children Have Died of Covid-19 in Gauteng as Hospital Admissions Drop'. *Times Live*, 10 September 2020. https://www.timeslive.co.za/news/south-africa/2020-09-10-35-children-have-died-of-covid-19-in-gauteng-as-hospital-admissions-drop/.
Njilo, Nonkululeko. '53% of Adults Want Schools Closed until Covid-19 Situation Improves – Survey'. *Times Live*, 13 January 2021. https://www.timeslive.co.za/news/south-africa/2021-01-13-53-of-adults-want-schools-closed-until-covid-19-situation-improves-survey/.
Ntshidi, Edwin. 'Gauteng Taxi Drivers Violate Lockdown Rules Despite Law Enforcement Presence'. *Eyewitness News*, 29 June 2020. https://ewn.co.za/2020/06/29/gauteng-taxi-drivers-violate-lockdown-rules-despite-law-enforcement-presence.
Nwachukwu, John Owen. 'Bill Gates Wonders Why Number of Covid-19 Cases, Deaths Are Not High in Africa'. *Daily Post*, 26 December 2020. https://dailypost.

ng/2020/12/26/bill-gates-wonders-why-number-of-covid-19-cases-deaths-are-not-high-in-africa/.

Parker, Alexandra, Gillian Maree, Graeme Gotz and Samkelisiwe Khanyile. 'How Covid-19 Puts Women at More Risk than Men in Gauteng, South Africa'. *The Conversation*, 21 December 2020. https://theconversation.com/how-covid-19-puts-women-at-more-risk-than-men-in-gauteng-south-africa-150570.

Paton, Carol. 'Business for SA Urges Urgent Opening of Economy to Avoid Jobs Bloodbath'. *Business Live*, 6 May 2020. https://www.businesslive.co.za/bd/national/2020-05-06-business-for-sa-urges-urgent-opening-of-economy-to-avoid-jobs-bloodbath/.

Patrick, Alex. 'Group of Leading Scientists Come out in Support of Glenda Gray Who Dared to Criticise Lockdown Rules'. *Times Live*, 23 May 2020. https://www.timeslive.co.za/news/south-africa/2020-05-23-group-of-leading-scientists-come-out-in-support-of-glenda-gray-who-dared-to-criticise-lockdown-regulations/.

Pijoos, Iavan. '"Beer Poured over His Head, Choked, Kicked, Hit with Machine Gun": How Collin Khosa Died in Alex'. *Times Live*, 15 April 2020. https://www.timeslive.co.za/news/south-africa/2020-04-15-beer-poured-over-his-head-choked-kicked-hit-with-machine-gun-how-collin-khosa-died-in-alex/.

Pijoos, Iavan. 'How to Protect Yourself from Airborne Transmission of Covid-19'. *Times Live*, 9 July 2020. https://www.timeslive.co.za/news/south-africa/2020-07-09-how-to-protect-yourself-from-airborne-transmission-of-covid-19/.

Pitjeng, Refilwe. 'Covid-19: What Exactly Is the National Command Council?' *Eyewitness News*, 4 May 2020.

Price, Max. 'Why Don't We Know How Many People Have Been Infected with Covid-19 in South Africa?' *Daily Maverick*, 5 May 2020. https://www.dailymaverick.co.za/article/2020-05-05-why-dont-we-know-how-many-people-have-been-infected-with-covid-19-in-south-africa.

Rawlinson, Kevin and Ian Sample. 'Oxford Covid Vaccine Has 10% Efficacy against South African Variant, Study Suggests'. *The Guardian*, 8 February 2021. https://www.theguardian.com/world/2021/feb/08/oxford-covid-vaccine-10-effective-south-african-variant-study.

Ray, Craig. 'Level 3 Regulations Edge SA Sports Federations to the Brink'. *Daily Maverick*, 1 June 2020. https://www.dailymaverick.co.za/article/2020-06-01-level-3-regulations-edge-sa-sports-federations-to-the-brink/.

Redaction Africanews. 'Protests Erupt in Senegal over New Covid-19 Measures'. *Africanews*, 7 January 2021. https://www.africanews.com/2021/01/07/protests-erupt-in-senegal-over-new-covid-19-measures/p. 148.

Rettner, Rachael. 'Instead of Just Flattening the Covid-19 Curve, Can We "Crush" it?' *Live Science*, 3 April 2020. https://www.livescience.com/can-covid-19-be-crushed.html.

Roy, Arundhati. 'We Are Witnessing a Crime against Humanity: Arundhati Roy on India's Covid Catastrophe'. *The Guardian*, 29 April 2021. https://www.theguardian.com/news/2021/apr/28/crime-against-humanity-arundhati-roy-india-covid-catastrophe.

SA News. 'New Committee to Focus on Covid-19 Vaccine for South Africa'. *Business Tech*, 15 September 2020. https://businesstech.co.za/news/trending/433571/new-committee-to-focus-on-covid-19-vaccine-for-south-africa/.

Savides, Matthew. 'Government "Ignored Expert Advice against Exceeding 70% Taxi Capacity"'. *Times Live*, 27 August 2020. https://www.timeslive.co.za/news/south-africa/2020-08-27-government-ignored-expert-advice-against-exceeding-70-taxi-capacity.

Schoub, Barry. 'The ABC of AstraZeneca Vaccine and the B.1.351 Variant'. *News24*, 23 March 2021. https://www.news24.com/news24/analysis/barry-schoub-the-abc-of-astrazeneca-vaccine-and-the-b1351-variant-20210323.

Seleka, Ntwaagae. 'Covid-19 Spike: Many Private Hospitals Full, Patients Sent to Public Hospitals – Health Minister'. *News24*, 29 December 2020. https://www.news24.com/news24/southafrica/news/covid-19-spike-many-private-hospitals-full-patients-sent-to-public-hospitals-health-minister-20201229.

Sguazzin, Antony and Pauline Bax. 'Where Are Our Coronavirus Vaccines? South Africans Ask'. *Bloomberg*, 21 January 2021. https://www.bloomberg.com/news/articles/2021-01-21/south-africa-s-vaccine-holdup-heaps-pressure-on-ramaphosa.

Shin, Hyonhee. 'South Korea to Tighten Social Distancing, Warns of New Covid-19 Crisis'. *Reuters*, 17 November 2020. https://www.reuters.com/article/us-health-coronavirus-southkorea-idUSKBN27W32M.

Smith, Elliot. 'South Africa Extends Lockdown but Offers Roadmap for Reopening'. *CNBC*, 15 April 2020. https://www.cnbc.com/2020/04/15/south-africa-extends-lockdown-but-offers-roadmap-for-reopening.html.

Smith, Emma. 'These Countries Have Only a Handful of Ventilators'. *Devex*, 9 April 2020. https://www.devex.com/news/these-countries-have-only-a-handful-of-ventilators-96970.

Sokutu, Brian. 'SA Has to "Learn from Asian Tigers" to Move Economy'. *The Citizen*, 29 August 2019. https://citizen.co.za/business/business-news/2172592/sa-has-to-learn-from-asian-tigers-to-move-economy/.

South African Broadcasting Corporation. 'Tembisa Hospital CEO to Face Suspension after Patient's Untimely Death'. *SABC News*, 30 January 2021. https://www.sabcnews.com/sabcnews/tembisa-hospital-ceo-to-face-suspension-after-patients-untimely-death/.

Soy, Anne. 'Lack of Covid-19 Testing Undermines Africa's "Success"'. British Broadcasting Corporation, 27 May 2020. https://www.bbc.com/news/world-africa-52801190.

Spinney, Laura. 'The Coronavirus Slayer! How Kerala's Rock Star Health Minister Helped Save it from Covid-19'. *The Guardian*, 14 May 2020. https://www.theguardian.com/world/2020/may/14/the-coronavirus-slayer-how-keralas-rock-star-health-minister-helped-save-it-from-covid-19.

Spinney, Laura. 'How Elimination Versus Suppression Became Covid's Cold War'. *The Guardian*, 3 March 2021. https://www.theguardian.com/commentisfree/2021/mar/03/covid-19-elimination-versus-suppression.

Sridhar, Devi. 'Crunching the Coronavirus Curve Is Better than Flattening it, as New Zealand Is Showing'. *The Guardian*, 22 April 2020. https://www.theguardian.com/commentisfree/2020/apr/22/flattening-curve-new-zealand-coronavirus.

Sridhar, Devi. 'As More Local Lockdowns Begin, the Hard Truth Is There's No Return to "Normal"'. *The Guardian*, 21 September 2020. https://www.theguardian.com/commentisfree/2020/sep/21/local-lockdowns-begin-no-normal-advice-live-with-covid.

Staff Reporter. 'Health Minister Names New Ministerial Advisory Committee on Social Change'. *Independent Online*, 17 June 2020. www.iol.co.za/news/politics/health-minister-names-new-advisory-committee-on-social-change-4943171.

Staff Writer. 'How Many South Africans Now Rely on Social Grants: 1996 vs 2020'. *BusinessTech*, 10 January 2021. https://businesstech.co.za/news/government/459186/how-many-south-africans-now-rely-on-social-grants-1996-vs-2020.

Staff Writer. 'Over 106,000 excess deaths reported in South Africa since first Covid-19 wave'. *BusinessTech*, 25 January 2021. https://businesstech.co.za/news/trending/463168/over-106000-excess-deaths-reported-in-south-africa-since-first-covid-19-wave/.

Stone, Setumo. 'Could This Handwashing Station be the Solution to SA's Hygiene Problems?' *City Press*, 1 June 2020. https://www.news24.com/citypress/news/could-this-handwashing-station-be-the-solution-to-sas-hygiene-problems-20200601.

Tandwa, Lizeka and Qaanita Hunter. 'Lockdown: Ramaphosa Lobbied to Open Places of Worship'. *News24*, 21 May 2020. https://www.news24.com/news24/SouthAfrica/News/lockdown-ramaphosa-lobbied-to-open-places-of-worship-20200521.

The Citizen. 'Medical Experts Slam Govt for Banning Booze but Loading Taxis'. 14 July 2020. https://citizen.co.za/news/covid-19/2320867/medical-experts-slam-govt-for-banning-booze-but-loading-taxis/.

TimesLive. 'Business Travel to be Phased in under level 3 – President Cyril Ramaphosa'. 24 May 2020. https://www.timeslive.co.za/politics/2020-05-24-business-travel-to-be-phased-in-under-level-3-president-cyril-ramaphosa/.

Tjiya, Emmanuel. 'Minister Ebrahim Patel Dictates to Fashion Police'. *Sowetan*, 14 May 2020. https://www.sowetanlive.co.za/entertainment/2020-05-14-minister-ebrahim-patel-dictates-to-fashion-police/.

Uys, Daniel and Schalk van der Merwe. 'Why Is the Covid-19 Mortality Rate so High in the Western Cape?' *Business Live*, 2 July 2020. https://www.businesslive.co.za/bd/opinion/2020-07-02-why-is-the-covid-19-mortality-rate-so-high-in-the-western-cape/.

Van der Merwe, Marelise. 'Some Businesses Will Reopen in May – but it Won't be Business as Usual'. *Fin24*, 23 April 2020. https://www.news24.com/fin24/economy/south-africa/some-businesses-will-reopen-but-it-wont-be-business-as-usual-20200423.

Van Onselen, Gareth. 'We Underestimated How Low Turnout Would Go – IRR'. *Politicsweb*, 12 May 2019. https://www.politicsweb.co.za/politics/postelection-poll-analysis—irr.

Wallis, William and Jasmine Cameron-Chileshe. 'UK Community Leaders Battle Vaccine Scepticism among Ethnic Minorities'. *Financial Times*, 1 February 2021. https://www.ft.com/content/9019eddf-6d65-4b8d-b7b3-241578dc6e4f.

Weismueller, Jason, Jacob Shapiro, Jan Oledan and Paul Harrigan. 'Coronavirus Misinformation Is a Global Issue, but which Myth You Fall for Likely Depends on Where You Live'. *The Conversation*, 11 August 2020. https://theconversation.com/coronavirus-misinformation-is-a-global-issue-but-which-myth-you-fall-for-likely-depends-on-where-you-live-143352.

White, Ray. 'Mbalula: Government Won't Tolerate Breaking of Lockdown Rules by Taxi Industry'. *Eyewitness News*, 16 July 2020. https://ewn.co.za/2020/07/16/govt-won-t-tolerate-breaking-of-lockdown-rules-by-taxi-industry-says-mbalula.

Winning, Alexander and Olivia Kumwenda-Mtambo. 'South Africa Puts AstraZeneca Vaccinations on Hold over Variant Data'. *Reuters*, 8 February 2021. https://www.reuters.com/article/uk-health-coronavirus-safrica-idUSKBN2A80J2.

INDEX

A
accountability 94, 112
   citizens 92, 113
   failure 102, 105, 128
   government/power 91–93, 100–101
   lack of 105
   lapse in 98
admissions *see* hospitals, admissions
Africa 1–24, 27, 39, 42–46, 49, 52, 88–89, 98, 121–124, 130–131
Africa CDC (Africa Centres for Disease Control and Prevention) 6, 9, 11, 39
Africa Centres for Disease Control and Prevention *see* Africa CDC
African National Congress (ANC) 63, 76, 96, 108–109, 121
African Population Health Research Centre 7
African Union 11
Afrikaans speakers 14
Afrikaners 14–15
age 7, 31, 37, 111
   profile 2
   school-going 35, 63, 67
   working 7, 37
Aids *see* HIV and Aids
alcohol 47–48
   ban 59, 81
   sales 47, 58, 81, 83, 89
Algeria 18
American Academy of Microbiology 46

American Institute for Economic Research (AIER) 35
ANC *see* African National Congress
Andersen, Kristian 36
anti-lockdown
   campaign 62
   lobbies 69, 84–85, 87
apartheid 13–17, 21, 23, 55, 67, 76, 105
   anti-apartheid 67
   cultural 15
   end of 128
   medical 63
   policy 96
   ravages of 115
   sporting 15
Association of American Physicians 46
Australasia 2
Australia 20, 52, 124, 130
authoritarian
   government 69
   rule/societies 92, 130
awareness 48, 80

B
Baker, Michael 39
Bank, Leslie 115, 120, 126, 130
Baragwanath *see* Chris Hani Baragwanath Academic Hospital
bars 25–26, 84
BBC *see* British Broadcasting Corporation

behaviour(s)
  citizens' 114
  correcting 92
  destructive 65
  necessary to avoid HIV 31
  patterns of 17
Bernault, Florence 42–43, 124
Bhekisisa Centre for Health
    Journalism 54
Biovac 27
black people 101
  admitted in subordinate positions 15
  becoming insiders 17–18, 20
  excluded from the vote and civil
    liberties 15
  forced to become citizens of
    independent statelets 13
  government by/rule by 16, 24
  incorporated into 'First World' on
    unequal terms 23
  more likely to be affected 101
  moved to suburbs 86
  provided with resources and
    opportunities 17
  rejection of the science 26
  sexual habits 28
  sharing cigarettes 47
Bolsonaro presidency (Brazil) 20
Brazil 3, 6, 20, 26, 41
  see also BRICS
BRICS (Brazil, Russia, India, China,
    South Africa) 4, 20, 109
British Broadcasting Corporation
    (BBC) 9–10, 45, 111, 115,
    121, 131
burial capacity 33
Business for South Africa 75–78
business travel 83–84
Business Unity South Africa 78

C
Canada 3, 20, 124
case and death
  numbers 36, 101, 122–125
  rate(s) 24, 130
  trajectory 84

case numbers 4, 10, 33, 43–44, 51–53, 72,
    81–82, 84, 94–97, 99, 107, 113, 127
  and deaths 11, 82, 114, 124–125, 128
  and fatalities 8, 56, 67
  and fatality rates 2
  hotspots 101
  South Africa's 1
cases and deaths 1–11, 14, 20, 34, 38,
    42, 50
  inevitable 72, 84, 99, 106
  keeping it down/low (reducing it) 53,
    82, 107, 122, 124, 128–129
  use test and trace to reduce 52
Charlotte Maxeke Johannesburg
    Academic Hospital 103
China 20, 33, 95, 122
  see also BRICS
Chris Hani Baragwanath Academic
    Hospital 63, 65, 70
cigarette(s) 47, 61, 78, 89
City Press 58–59
climate 2
climate change 35
  conference (COP17) 123
clinics 116
clothing
  regulations 63
  sales 61
Coetzee, Ryan 59–60
colonial prejudices 115
colonialism 14
colonisers 17–18
coloured people 87, 96
comorbidities 35, 63, 67
competence 21, 129, 131
Conference of Parties (COP17) 123
The Conversation 50
cooked food 47, 58
Coovadia, Cas 78
corticosteroids 103
Covid/Covid-19
  dashboard 7
  limiting the effect 1
  'long Covid' 6, 37
  modelling 29
  Modelling Consortium 27

prevention measures 116
regulations 88
research 55
response to 4, 24, 26, 28–29, 33, 40, 87, 89, 93, 103, 129, 131–132
rules 48
scientific consensus 86
severe 50–51
technological responses 104–105
Cronje, Frans 60
crowded/overcrowded
    conditions 8
    dwellings/homes 49, 128
    taxis 116, 128
    township houses/shacks 19
Cuba 23
cultural
    apartheid 15
    divide 24
    priorities of the suburbs 88
curative
    health assets 42
    medicine 41–44, 50, 55, 94, 98–99, 108, 123, 130–131
    model 121
curve (of infections) 33, 39, 45, 51, 53, 127
customary gatherings 116
customary practices 115

D
DA *see* Democratic Alliance
Dasoo, Aslam 62–64, 67–68, 70, 72, 81, 107
deaths 1, 6–11, 14, 23, 44, 73, 93, 96
    see also case numbers; case and death; cases and deaths; illnesses and deaths
    and hospitalisations 34, 45
    excess deaths 34, 104
    reducing 104, 127
defeatism 123, 128
democracy 68, 92, 127, 130
    power accountability 91, 101, 128
    South Africa 13, 19, 23, 98

Democratic Alliance (DA) 60, 86, 96, 106, 108
denialism (HIV and Aids) 28–29
deracialising the economy and universities 17
dexamethasone 104
digital media 3, 19, 61, 67, 88, 91, 100, 102
distancing 29, 48, 51, 114, 116
Dlamini Zuma, Nkosazana 26, 47, 61
domestic consumer markets 94
domestic history 27
domestic politics 20

E
East Asia 1–2, 52, 82, 121
East Asian countries 42, 44
East Asian 'tigers' 124
Eastern Cape 72, 84, 114–115, 117, 120, 126
Ebola 42, 98
economic
    activity 64
    activity back on track 60
    activity restricted/curtailed/obstructed 25, 37, 57
    bargaining 20
    challenges 132
    compromises 20
    considerations 26
    constraint 37, 61
    cost of lockdown 78, 97
    exclusion 94
    gains reversed 64
    hardship 59
    impact of pandemic 8
    interests of 'anti-scientists' 25
    life constraint/suspension 31, 37
    power 23
    priorities of the suburbs 88
    recovery 79
    restrictions 25
Economic Intervention work group 76
economy
    deracialising 17

economy (*continued*)
   formal 18–19
   hampered by health measures 54
   health of market economy 76
   participation 18, 22
   reopening 77–79
elderly 7, 35, 63, 67, 114
English-speakers 14
Europe 6, 14, 17, 20, 50
excess deaths 34, 104, 119

F
fatalities/fatality 6, 8, 68, 88
   figures/numbers 4, 7, 56
   in intensive care 104
   Nordic 36
   rate(s) 2, 5, 73
   trends 84
   UK 36
Fauci, Anthony 52
first wave 11, 52, 104, 115, 127
First World 19, 21–24, 37, 55, 58, 61–62, 66, 71–76, 79, 83–89, 94–101, 104–108, 111–112, 115, 117, 120, 122–123, 128–131
   citizens 61
   excellence 71
   health care facilities 43
   medicine 50
   minority 56
   scientists 66
   thinking 87
   vision 38–49
following the science 25–56, 81, 83–84, 87, 113, 128
food
   access to 66
   cooked 47, 58
   means to store 64, 69
   parcels 48
   running out of money for 8
France 40
funerals 115–116

G
Garden Route 72, 114
Gates, Bill 10
Gauteng City-Region Observatory (GCRO) 7
Gauteng Visual Analytics Platform 101
GCRO *see* Gauteng City-Region Observatory
gender 7
   -based violence 22, 80
   composition 61
Germany 14, 20, 124
Ghebreyesus, Tedros Adhanom 45
Gray, Glenda 34–38, 62–73, 82, 85–86, 99, 106–108, 114
Great Barrington Declaration 35, 37, 52, 67
Groote Schuur Hospital 34, 41, 105

H
Habib, Adam 65
health-care
   decision-making 63
   facilities 2, 43, 51
   workers 50
health facilities 3–4, 74, 117
Heneghan, Carl 52
herd immunity 35–36, 38
Heywood, Mark 66
HIV and Aids 27–29, 31, 34, 37, 43, 54–55, 72, 115
   denialism 28–29
Hofmeyr, Ross 41
hospitalisations 34, 45, 50
hospitals 19, 42–43, 65, 85, 117
   admissions 10, 38, 96, 102, 104
   closure 116
   effectiveness of care 102–103
   Gauteng 104
   malnutrition at public hospitals 99
   overwhelming 125
   pressure 48, 94
   reality 78
   state of 115
   treatment impact 41

Index

HSRC *see* Human Sciences Research Council
human behaviour 32
Human Sciences Research Council (HSRC) 86, 115
humanities 32

I

ignorance 21, 24
  of mental health 48
illnesses and deaths 54, 93, 127
incapacity 10, 21, 24, 115, 117
incompetence 10, 21, 88, 96, 121
India 3, 6, 20, 44, 122
  see also BRICS
  Kerala 44, 122
  Serum Institute of India 112
Indian people 87
Indonesia 43
infection(s)
  acceptable level 107
  driving down 82
  high levels/rates 48, 96, 101, 127
  increase/rising 83, 95, 97, 113, 116, 120, 125
  mass 69
  preventing 33–34, 42
  second wave 4, 72, 81, 86, 94, 104
  slowing the rate 74
  spreading 29
  surge 75
  third wave 114
initiation schools 116
insider(s) 17–23, 58, 79, 92, 98, 100–101, 129
interest group politics 81, 88
interest groups 24, 75, 81
International Monetary Fund (IMF) 79
Ireland 20
Italy 40, 42

J

Joint United Nations Programme on HIV/AIDS (UNAIDS) Scientific Expert Panel 46

journalism 100
journalists 69, 99–100, 105, 109, 131

K

Karim, Salim Abdool 3, 9–10, 27–28, 33, 38–39, 45, 49, 54, 62, 64–66, 72, 82–84, 95–99, 114, 119
Kekana, Mahlamola 85–86
Kenya 7, 18
Khosa, Collins 47

L

The Lancet 130
Latin America 6, 9, 14, 82, 130
Lethole, Shonisani 102–103
liberation politics 24
living
  conditions 2
  in confinement 59
  in households with pre-existing conditions 8
  in poverty 9, 20, 40, 48–49, 54, 68, 91, 97, 106, 113–114
  with children 8
lobbies/lobbying 87–89
  anti-common-sense 31
  anti-lockdown 84–85, 87–88
  anti-restriction(s) 88–89, 127
  business 92
  by interest groups 75, 81
  for the removal of restrictions 77
  government's response 82
  power and influence 83
  relaxation of regulations 81, 84
  religious 80, 92
  scientists 92
  sport 80
  surrender to 125
  taxi industry 85
  to lock down early 39
  to reopen economy/enterprises 77–79
lockdown 8, 33–39, 45, 47, 51–88, 93–101, 106, 108, 113, 124–125, 129
  denounced/denouncing 39, 49, 75
  ending it 52
  harsher 51

179

lockdown (*continued*)
    legal action 60
    levels 58
    opponents/opposition 53, 72
    rejection 60
    restrictions 116
    support dropping 58
'long Covid' 6, 37
Lysenko/Lysenkoism 28

M
MAC *see* Ministerial Advisory Committee
macroeconomic analysis 77
Madhi, Shabir 9–10, 34, 38, 45, 50, 52, 62, 70, 81, 95, 98–99, 107, 110–112
Makgoba, Malegapuru 102
Malan, Mia 54–55, 62
malnutrition 68
    at Baragwanath 63, 65, 70
    at public hospitals 99
    in Soweto 106
Mandela, Nelson 16
masks 25, 30–32, 48
    wearing 30, 51, 114
Matshiqi, Aubrey 19
Mauritius 20
Mbalula, Fikile 85
Mbeki, Thabo 16, 27–29
media 24, 66
    British 115, 124
    broadcast 119
    conferences 99–100
    coverage of township areas 48
    digital/social 3, 19, 61, 67, 88, 100, 102
    exposed Zuma 127
    financial 76–78
    holding power to account 100–101
    in the global North 9
    indifference to Africa 3
    industry 101
    international 108
    platform for scientists 24
    South African 3, 100
    uncritical coverage 112

    Western 3, 20
medical apartheid 63
medical science 32, 82, 104
    abuse by 26
medical scientists 9, 25, 27, 32–34, 52, 56, 67, 69, 71, 87
    accountability/responsibility 98
    advised restricting taxis 85
    Africa's 11
    denouncing government for not buying vaccines early 107
    denouncing lockdown 81
    disputes 55
    influence of 88
    South African 10, 33, 41, 43–44, 50, 53
    sweeping statements 83
Mendelson, Marc 34, 38, 50, 53, 62–63, 69–70, 81, 95, 98–99
Mer, Mervyn 103
Mexico 5–6
Meyer, Piet 14
militarising control of the virus 68
military's role in policing the rules 47
Ministerial Advisory Committee (MAC) 3, 27–28, 32–33, 54, 62, 64–66, 111
minority rule 4, 68, 105, 131
Mkhize, Zweli 7, 11, 27–28, 38, 64–66, 69, 72–74, 81, 104, 115, 119
modern medicine 43
Moderna pharmaceutical company 109
modernity 20, 43, 95–96
Modi government (India) 20
Morocco 119–120

N
Namibia 18
National Association of Parents in School Governance 85–86
National Blood Service 101
National Coronavirus Command Council (NCCC) 26–27, 74
National Income Dynamics Study-Coronavirus Rapid Mobile Survey (NIDS-CRAM) 7–8

National Institute for Communicable
   Diseases (NICD) 27
National Institute of Allergy and
   Infectious Diseases (USA) 52
Nature 10, 45
NCCC *see* National Coronavirus
   Command Council
NICD *see* National Institute for
   Communicable Diseases
Nicolaou, Stavros 78
Nigeria 8, 20, 120
Nel, Daan de Wet 15
New Zealand 1, 39, 44, 52, 82, 107, 121,
   130
Nkengasong, John 11, 39
North America (United States and
   Canada) 3–4, 18, 20, 44
   centrality 24
   dominant culture 14

O
O'Donnell, Guillermo 130
outsiders 17, 19, 21–22, 129
Oxford University 30
oxygen 41, 102

P
Patel, Ebrahim 47, 74
Paterson, Mark 115
Pillay, Anban 65, 70
policy
   and the public debate 129
   apartheid 96
   debate 20, 22
   foreign 23
   government 15, 76
   preference 85
   public 4
political
   challenges 132
   class 24
   considerations 26
   interference 68
   leadership of black majority 76
   life 19
   majority 19

minority 19
parties 88, 101
perspective 20
processes 83
right 37
scientists 88
politicians 16, 63
   elected 87
   'First World' 24
politics 29
   and policy debate 22
   domestic 20
   'First World' 101
   insider 22, 101
   interest group 81, 88
   liberation politics 24
polling 60–61
poverty 13, 17, 20–21, 40, 105,
      126, 129
   Latin America 9
   of vision/vision of 46–49
   people living in 9, 20, 40, 48–49,
      54, 68, 91, 97, 106, 113–114,
      126
power 22, 68, 70, 131
   access to 24
   accountability 91–93, 100–101, 114,
      128
   and influence of lobbies 83
   bargaining 109
   challengers of 70
   corridors of 88
   economic 23
   holders of 92–93, 114
   losing (Zuma) 127
   of command council 68
   of lobbies 83
   of taxi industry 85
   supernatural 74
   to influence a debate 22–23
   wealthy countries' bargaining 109
   which created the curative medicine
      131
prejudice(s)
   about lifestyles and cultures 21
   colonial 115

prejudice(s) (*continued*)
   First World 72, 115
   science a euphemism for 31
   suburban 67
   white 16
prescience 120, 123
preventative/preventive
   health capacity 45
   measures 33, 42, 120
   medicine 43, 121
   strategies 29, 42, 121
preventing
   disease among older people 31
   health facilities/hospitals from being overwhelmed 74, 125
   infections 33–34, 42
   outbreaks of irresponsibility 47
   people engaging in drunken violence 47
   people smoking 47
   people wandering in public 47
   the virus spreading 25, 97
prevention 42
   management 50
   measures 116
   response 113
price/pricing
   of doses 109
   of ventilators 77
priorities/priority
   business concerns 80
   containment 110
   government's 16
   health of citizens 26
   of interests 24
   of organised sport 80
   of scientists 39
   of the insiders 22
   of the suburbs 88
   public health 122
   the country's 24
   to preserve health and life 54, 122–123
   to ready the health system 43
   to testing and tracing 52
   Progressive Health Forum 62

protection 30, 110, 127
protective
   equipment 75
   factor 34
   measures 25, 31, 40, 72, 85
public health 122
   emergency 63
   knowledge 124
   measures 29, 42, 54, 108
   protecting 69
   response 74–75
   skills 131
   system 40, 43
   techniques 128
public health care services 8

R
racial
   barriers 17
   composition 18, 61
   divide about opening schools 86
   divisions 23
   minorities 87
   minority rule *see* minority rule
   policies 76
   separation 15
Ramaphosa, Cyril 23, 59, 61, 74–76, 80, 83, 97, 113
   enthusiasm for science 28
   government's response 28
Rapport 58
relief package 59, 77
religious
   activity/life 25, 31
   leaders 80, 88
   lobbies 80, 92
   services 26, 81, 83
resources
   access to 24
   available among South Africans 115
   available to the country 122
   providing black people with 17
   to influence a debate 22
restaurants 26, 48, 78, 80–81, 84
restricting
   activity 26, 108

taxis 85
restriction(s) 47–48, 68–69, 73, 84, 86–87, 93, 95
   anti-restriction lobby 88–89, 127
   credibility 106
   damage caused 79, 92
   easing/lifting/reducing/relaxing 59, 61, 75, 77, 79, 81–83, 88, 95, 97, 113, 125
   economic and social life 25, 37
   ending 100
   extended 58
   imposing 28, 127
   increase/tighten 53, 113
   lockdown 116
   need for 31
   opponents/opposition to 34, 53
   refusal to impose 114
   religious activity 25
   retain 125
   severe 58
   to flatten the curve/ready the health system/slow the spread 39, 47
   travel 116
   unscientific 35
restrictive measures 53
Rhodes Must Fall 17
risk adjusted approach/strategy 28, 58, 64, 81, 83
rural 120
   funerals 115
   life 116
   people/population 120–121
   poor 116, 121
Russia(ns) 6, 110
   see also BRICS
   vaccines 109–110

S
SADC *see* Southern African Development Community
Sage *see* Scientific Advisory Group for Emergencies
SAHPRA *see* South African Health Products Regulatory Authority
SAIRR *see* South African Institute of Race Relations
SAMRC *see* South African Medical Research Council
Sanne, Ian 64
school(s) 126
   in Britain 67
   closed 64, 69, 85
   initiation 116
   open/reopen 48, 67, 85–86, 88
   principals 126
   suburban 19
school-going children 35, 63, 67
schooling 19, 106
science
   following *see* following the science
   medical *see* medical science
   of the suburbs 62–75
   social 32, 43
   unravels 57–89
Scientific Advisory Group for Emergencies (Sage) 44
screening and testing 28, 49, 64
Scripps Research Institute (La Jolla, California) 36
second wave 1, 82, 107
   Africa 11
   Britain 36
   India 3, 6, 44
   South Africa 4, 6, 72, 81, 86, 94, 99–100, 104, 113–117, 119, 125, 129
Section 27 41
Serum Institute of India 112
shacks/shack settlement 21, 46, 73, 97, 106, 127, 129, 131
   burden of Covid 93
   government engagement 49
   supporting restrictions 87
Sharpley, Nelly Vuyokazi 115
SIR model 30
Skweyiya, Zola 126
smoking 47, 61–62
social
   activity restrictions/suspension 25, 31
   and behavioural change committee 25

social (continued)
  campaigns 22
  challenges 132
  development 126
  distancing *see* distancing
  grants 21–22, 126
  impact of the pandemic 8
  media *see* digital media
  networks 117
  processes 83
  sciences 32, 43
  scientists 65
socialists 79
society
  burden of 128–132
  capacity of 123
  'First World' 89
  influential voices 16
  knowledge of 32
  suburban 17
socioeconomic challenges 59
Somalia 9
sophistication 20–21, 43, 48, 72, 95–96
South African Health Products Regulatory Authority (SAHPRA) 110
South African Institute of Race Relations (SAIRR) 60
South African Medical Journal 32, 50
South African Medical Research Council (SAMRC) 27, 34, 65–66, 104
South Korea 33, 40, 42, 52, 107, 121–122, 124, 130
Southern African Development Community (SADC) 7
Soweto 68, 106
Spinney, Laura 38–39, 54–55
sport 80
sporting
  apartheid 15
  events 58, 123
  industry 81
Stalin, Joseph 28
Street, Alice 43, 97

suburban
  concerns about government 106
  consensus 76
  enraged opinion 47
  lifestyle 55
  middle class 66
  prejudice 67
  residents 20, 48, 106
  schools 19
  sentiment 69
  society 17
  view of the world 67
suburbanites 47–48, 67–68
suburbs 13, 15, 20–21, 37, 48, 61, 86–88, 93–94, 96–97, 101, 113, 129
  on the march 75–81
  priorities 88
  restrictions 58
  the science of 62–75
support and relief packages 77
Sweden 20, 35–36
Switzerland 31

T

Taiwan 72, 122, 124, 130
taverns 47, 116
taxis 46, 48, 66, 85, 87
  overcrowding 49, 116, 128
  powerful lobby 85
  restricting 85
TB (tuberculosis) 34
Tembisa Hospital 102–103
testing/tests 6–11, 28, 36–37, 39, 49, 73, 96–97
  and screening 28, 49, 64
  and tracing 49–54, 95–99, 101, 114–115, 125, 127–128
  backing up in the national laboratory 97–98
  failure 95, 97
  sign of 'sophistication' and modernity 95
  strategy 64
third wave 113–114
Third World 21, 23–24, 41, 46–48, 55–56, 58, 61, 66, 71, 79,

Index

93–94, 105, 11–112, 115, 126, 128–131
   majority 23, 56, 85
   victims of heavy-handed lockdown enforcement 106
Time magazine 13
tobacco sales 47, 58–59, 61, 83
township(s) 21, 46, 49, 68, 73, 87, 93, 97, 101, 105–106, 126–127, 129, 131
   abiding by the rules 47–48
   Alexandra 47
   attitudes 48
   crowded houses/shacks 19
   housing and schooling 106
   irresponsibility 47
   staying out of hospital and alive 85
   supporting restrictions 87
tracing 97–99, 126
   see also testing and tracing
Trade and Industry Policy Strategies 84
traditional ceremonies 116
traditional healers 117, 121, 126
traditional herbs and remedies 116
traditional leaders 121
transport 85
   public 8
   taxis 46
travel/travelling
   between provinces 116
   business *see* business travel
   in taxis 85
   restrictions 116
Treatment Action Campaign 41
Trump, Donald 96
   administration 37
   White House 35
Tshabalala-Msimang, Manto 29
tuberculosis (TB) 34
Turner, Richard 14

U

UK *see* United Kingdom
UNAIDS *see* Joint United Nations Programme on HIV/AIDS
United Kingdom (UK) 35–36, 40–41, 55, 96, 108, 115
   advisors/experts 44
   scientists 45
United States of America (USA) 3, 6, 9, 20, 26, 35–36, 40, 44, 50, 55, 81–82, 84, 96, 129, 132
   National Institute of Allergy and Infectious Diseases 52
University of Cape Town 27
University of Johannesburg 86
University of Stellenbosch 27
University of the Witwatersrand (Wits) 9, 27, 34, 52, 65
urban congestion 115
US National Academy of Medicine 46

V

vaccine(s) 26–27, 30–32, 36, 44, 94, 100, 108, 131
   approved 31, 107–108
   AstraZeneca 30, 110–111
   buying/procurement/securing 99, 107, 109–110, 112–113, 125
   Chinese 109–110
   discovery 4
   Johnson & Johnson 107–108, 111
   manufacture 27
   roll out 107, 113
   Russian 109–110
   sharing 10
   withdrawing 31, 113
Van Onselen, Gareth 60
ventilation 85
   mechanical 41
ventilators 41, 75, 77, 102–103, 105
   acquisition 103
Victory Research 59–60
violence
   against women 23
   by soldiers 106
   drunken 47
   fuelled by alcohol 48
   gender-based 22, 80
vulnerabilities 35
vulnerable 35, 63, 67, 106
   categories 37
   communities 49

W
Walter Sisulu University 115
Western Cape 72, 84, 96–97, 114–115
western civilisation 14
Western Europe 3–4, 10, 14, 18, 20, 24, 44, 82, 84, 129, 132
   governments 122
white
   Afrikaans speakers 14
   Afrikaners 15
   angst 18
   areas 14
   citizens 16
   -collar jobs 15
   domination 13
   emigration 18
   employers 15
   liberals 14
   life patterns 21
   people 18–19, 21, 96, 101
   prejudices 16
   right-wing politicians 15
   rule 14, 16, 18
   settlement 17
   South Africa(ns) 14, 62, 96
   world 15
Winde, Alan 97, 114
Wood, Robin 99
World Cup 58, 123
   2010 football 58, 123
World Health Organization (WHO) 5, 7, 11, 39, 44–46, 54, 81, 110, 124
WHO *see* World Health Organization
Wits *see* University of the Witwatersrand

Z
Zimbabwe 18
Zuma, Jacob 127

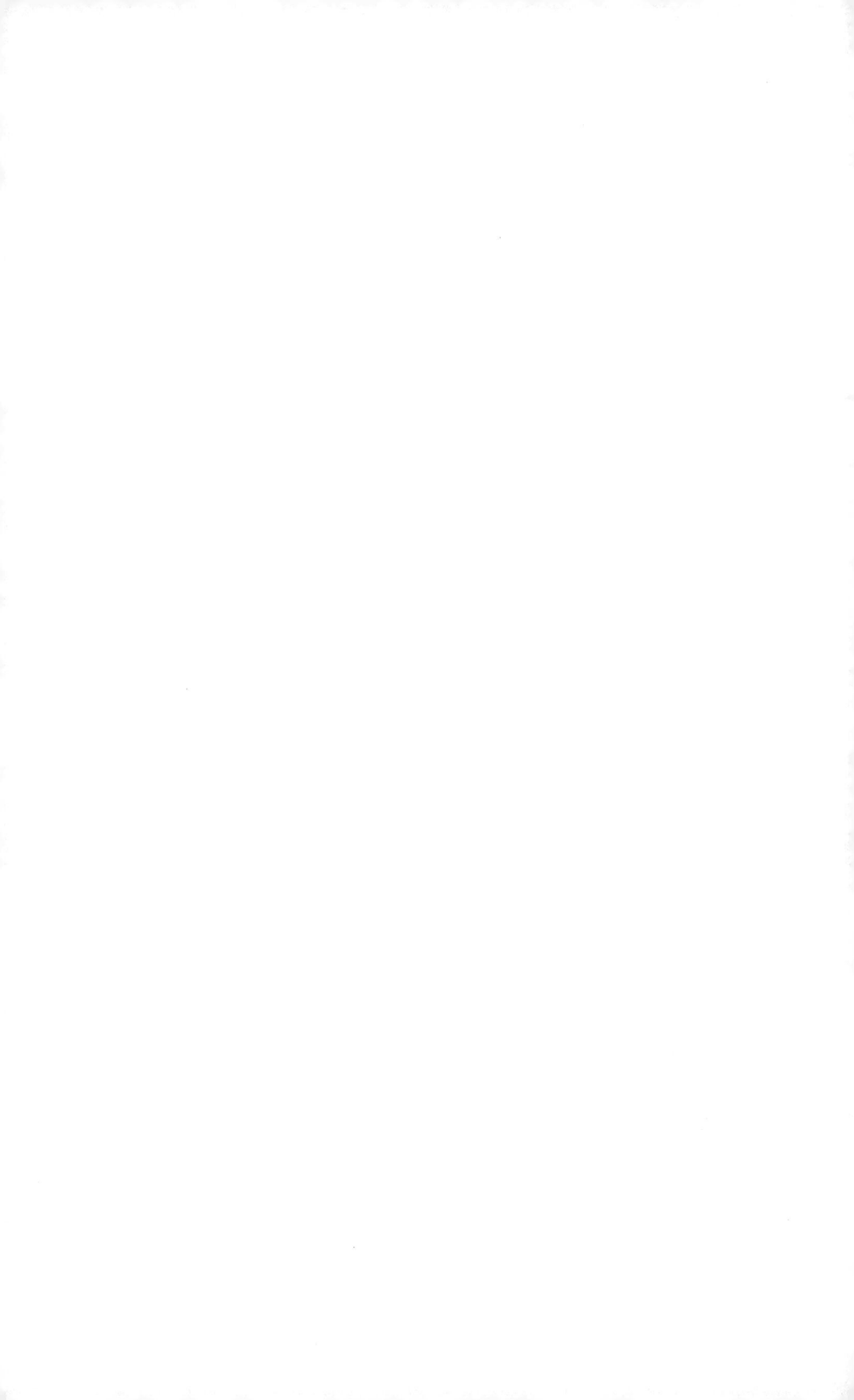

Lightning Source UK Ltd.
Milton Keynes UK
UKHW012008181121
394147UK00001B/47